Relationships in the NHS

This book is dedicated to our best relationships:
with Patricia and Phillippa;
without which it would not have been possible.

Relationships in the NHS
Bridging the Gap

Geoff Meads
Professor of Health Services Development
Health Management Group
City University, London, UK

and

John Ashcroft
Research Director
Relationships Foundation
Cambridge, UK

A Relationships Foundation Project based on emerging primary care organizations in conjunction with the Health Management Group, City University, London

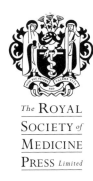

The ROYAL
SOCIETY of
MEDICINE
PRESS Limited

British Library Cataloguing in Publication Data
A catalogue record for this book is available from the British Library

ISBN: 1-85315-438-5

Phototypeset by Saxon Graphics Ltd, Derby

Printed in Great Britain by Bell & Bain Ltd, Glasgow

Contents

Forewords
Gillian Morgan
Michael Schluter

Foreword

The Government is committed to modernising public services. This requires better integration between organizations in both policy formulation and service delivery. The rhetoric of competition has been replaced by emphasis on co-operation and partnership. Making this real will require effective relationships at both organizational and personal levels. In parallel with the policy shift, structural changes are increasing the range and complexity of relationships. New organizations are being formed, for example, primary care groups and trusts, whilst other familiar organizations are likely to disappear. This will change the dynamics of the healthcare system and increase ambiguity and uncertainty.

The new agenda requires everyone working in the NHS including clinicians, managers and policy makers, to develop a better understanding of how organizations relate most effectively. The importance of improving relationships is frequently neglected although the characteristics of effective partnerships are well documented. Understanding of respective roles, shared purpose, trust and respect are essential if confidence is to be generated. These do not occur by chance and require time and effort to develop and sustain. Effective partnerships offer real benefits in a time of limited resources but too often these are not realised.

This book looks at the characteristics of NHS relationships. It looks at policy and the theory underpinning these relationships and builds on practical examples from many of the health communities in England. It offers new insights to those of us who are trying to harness and focus the energies of different organizations for the greater benefit of the populations that we serve.

Dr Gillian Morgan
Chief Executive
North & East Devon Health Authority

Foreword

Partnership, collaboration, involvement, 'joined-up' government: the language of relationships pervades current health policy and practice. The complexity and uniqueness of any relationship means that the reality of this rhetoric must involve more than motherhood and apple pie. Yet healthcare has always been about relationships – between health professionals and patients, between the health professions, or between purchasers and providers. So why the greater and more explicit attention to relationships now? Is this just window-dressing with warm language or does it represent a significant cultural shift? This book powerfully argues that there has been a significant culture shift in the NHS, and that the gap between Government rhetoric and relational reality must not be ignored.

The reasons for the greater attention being devoted to relationships lie in part outside the NHS, for concern about relationships can be seen across public and private sector organizations, and indeed across society as a whole. In our work at the Relationships Foundation we have found expressions of this concern in areas of public life as diverse as criminal justice, urban regeneration, welfare provision and business strategy. So why this concern? In part, it is rooted in growing recognition of the importance of relationships for individuals, communities and organizations. Relationships are central to individual well-being: they affect our health; shape our identity and sense of belonging; are a significant factor in our physical, financial and emotional security. Organizations, too, are increasingly aware of the importance of relationships whether as part of their service delivery, their strategic priorities, their capacity to innovate or their underlying efficiency and profitability.

More negatively, the interest in relationships is a reflection of their perceived weakness in contemporary Britain, the pressures they are under and the costs and consequences of their dysfunction. The importance of the relational well-being of individuals is the backdrop to the growing public concern about social exclusion, particularly for lonely, elderly people and the long-term unemployed. The pressure on relationships in our society is also showing itself in households and communities. Many families are struggling, as evidenced by high divorce rates and the growing need for parenting support. Poor town planning, high levels of population mobility, patterns of commuting and a culture of privacy have weakened many communities.

While the resilience of relationships and their capacity to adapt to social and cultural change should not be underestimated, the consequences of these relational stresses in terms of health, educational attainment and the happiness of individuals cannot be ignored. These personal experiences of relationship difficulties in family and community life spill over into the workplace. The organizational and professional relationships of the NHS are profoundly influenced by these trends, and in turn impact on them.

In addition to problems in families and communities there are other factors within the wider social environment which are bringing pressure to bear on relationships in both public and private life. These include the impact of new information and communication technologies which mean that the time we have for relationships is spread ever more thinly across a wider and wider network of friends and contacts. Also, the rising tide of individualism and materialism upsets the balance between rights and obligations, and devalues traditions such as mealtimes that provide the context for relationships to deepen and flourish. The desire for altruistic and committed relationships may be widespread, but for many people, both personally and professionally, they remain elusive.

The challenge of relational healthcare, however, goes beyond simply trying to ensure that effective relationships are maintained despite the pressures on them. This book is, therefore, more than just a useful guide to bridging the gap between rhetoric and practice. A focus on relationships is likely to challenge assumptions, behaviours, values and priorities. The authors set out a vision of what healthcare, particularly primary healthcare, could become if the ambiguities and ambivalence of the current transition period are resolved. They explore how a relational approach involves rethinking all the core functions of an organization from policy making through to performance review.

I believe a focus on relationships can be re-integrating, providing a shared agenda for fragmented services. It can also be inspiring: just as the morale of many health professionals has been undermined by negative experience of healthcare relationships, so too the prospect of renewed relationships has unlocked new energy and commitment. But without transformation of organizational culture and working practices, there is a risk that recent changes in NHS structures to achieve a much needed shift of focus will lead to cynicism, resentment and a collapse of the high delivery standards which we have in the past, too often taken for granted.

I hope this book will be widely read, and that reflection on its message will lead to fundamental and widespread changes in management styles, working practices, education and training to allow the new structures to live up to their undoubtedly great potential.

Michael Schluter
Director
The Relationships Foundation

Preface

The NHS has a particular interest in relationships. Those of the right sort contribute to health. Those of the wrong kind inhibit its capacity to plan and provide healthcare. The contemporary NHS, as it translates itself from a traditional bureaucratic institution into a modern healthcare system, commits a great deal of time, energy and attention to the structuring and restructuring of its relationships. These now encompass the independent sector – private, voluntary, commercial and consumerist – in ways that could hardly have been envisaged just a decade ago. The NHS is no longer just its staff and its patients. The past 10 years have witnessed the demise of over 400 statutory healthcare organizations. There have been no fewer than four separate NHS Acts approved by Parliament, and the next seems likely to confirm that up to 90% of public NHS resources will be directly controlled by groups of primary care professionals. General Medical Practitioners, in other words, will be the pivotal point for virtually all relationships throughout both the NHS and the UK healthcare system.

It is the new context for relationships that this book seeks to address. Rather like general practice its message is both old and new; endeavouring to adapt to rapidly changing circumstances while maintaining what is fundamental. Many of tomorrow's GPs, after all, will have to learn commissioning skills to add to their clinical toolkits. They will have to operate in larger groups or even out of alternative primary care organizations. But they will still be independent contractors steadfastly serving individual patients on their registered lists. Their relationship will remain that of an essential intermediary between the state and the individual, semi-detached from both, and the medium through which the basic dynamic which fuses collaborative and personal responsibilities for health and healthcare finds much of its expression.

This relationship is, accordingly, both a constant and a change agent. Other parts of the NHS, as well as general practice, also have a particular relational significance. Community hospitals can often help encapsulate rural identities, especially when under threat of survival. The hospital itself, as both a conceptual and capital construct, has oscillated over the past century between a focus on locally geographic areas and a specialist emphasis, reflecting very often the changing balance between popular and professional interest groups. The different components of the NHS do not simply help to make up a healthcare system; they also contribute significantly to the relational fabric of society itself.

The interaction between this system and society during the 1990s has been characterized by what many have felt personally and profoundly to be a growing dissonance between values and behaviour. Depending upon the different political positions of individuals, the original founding values of the NHS – free, equal and universal – have been progressively either augmented or circumvented. *Equal* has become *equitable* or even e*quivalent* and these changing values have been applied to formulae for resource allocation rather than service levels or healthcare outcomes. Financial charging has increased for general dental services, prescriptions, nursing homes and eye tests, for example. The mixed economy of care today means using a range of alternative funding mechanisms of which the Private Finance Initiative is merely the most publicly visible because of its associations with large hospital buildings. *Universal* has shifted subtly towards targets for *comprehensive* coverage – something quite different – on the back of which a new diversity of organizational types has been legitimized. The standard model general practice or district general hospital are already things of the past. By May 1997 – the pivotal moment for the action research on which this book is based – espoused and expressed NHS values had become distant relations in many parts of the country.

The new Labour administration that was elected at this time was firmly committed to the reassertion of core NHS values. It also recognized the need to preserve the performance benefits of its predecessor's healthcare reforms. Reconciling these two pragmatic imperatives has been a major political challenge. The first has meant seeking to reintegrate the contemporary NHS through process, to emphasize evolution and to eschew another early round of organizational re-engineering. *Cooperation* and *integration* have been the hallmark values propagated, for example, through cross-sectoral healthcare programmes, inter-practice commissioning groups and the revival of locally representative committees and boards. The second imperative of maintaining the enhanced efficiency of the NHS through an effective combination of local incentives and penalties (but without preserving GP fundholding-style market competition), has meant further moves towards total resource management at local levels, albeit within strengthened national frameworks for decision making in such areas as clinical effectiveness, prescribing and professional development.

Together these two imperatives can properly be understood as providing a revised paradigm for relationships in the UK healthcare system based upon the principles of *partnership* and *decentralization*. They sound good. The NHS generally feels better. The public is more optimistic. Only the performance indicators sometimes tell a different story: trusts in debt; waiting lists and times high and, in places, climbing; bed shortages for severely mentally ill people in London and bed blockages for frail elderly patients elsewhere. Espousing the right values does not automatically make everything better. Indeed, reviving liberal concepts without at least retaining the residual benefits of too readily discarded rightist philosophies can actually make things worse and be counterproductive. There are many applied academics around who quite plausibly argue that the 1991–96 NHS internal market was itself merely a pilot: now being evaluated prior to its more pervasive and enduring rehabilitation at the heart of the future UK healthcare system in the 21st century. The relationships challenge of new Labour's 'new NHS' is nothing if not real.

Aspects of this challenge are as old as the NHS (and in some cases older): seeking more effective collaboration between organizations and medical professions, for example, is not a new agenda. But the 'New NHS' does also present new challenges:

for GPs, for example, this may include a four-fold multiplication of the number of relationships with all their potential for competing demands and loyalties; conflicting models of relationship, (what, for example, is the appropriate model for leadership in the new NHS?), and an environment which can put relationships under extreme pressure. In taking on this challenge directly this book addresses the core functions of a health service from a relational perspective. Each function has its own relationships challenges; each depends upon relationships for effective operation. But relationships are not just a means, they are an important part of the definition of the end. Thus, when viewed from a relational perspective, each function must also be reinterpreted as well as pursued differently. An underlying theme has been a basic four-fold framework for healthcare relationships: caring, collaborative, competitive, convergent. This typology provides the book's subtext. More importantly, it also supplies the recognition that, for example, both competitive and collaborative relational styles may be appropriate and justifiable within the contemporary healthcare system so long as their contingent expression is rooted in a sound basic structure for relationships.

One common response to the relationships challenge of the legacy of the internal market and the promotion of a 'New NHS' has been a desire to restore the relationships of the past. But the snake was in that garden too. What the new NHS will prove to be is uncertain, not least with regard to its relationships. It will need wise leadership to look to the future and nurture new and fragile relationships through a transitional process which will, at times, be difficult. In this project we have tried to capture the experience, the learning and indeed the wisdom of many project participants. Wiser authors might have suspended judgement until the future was clearer, but that would not help those who have to work today with the ambiguities and ambivalence of an NHS in transition.

Geoff Meads
John Ashcroft
November 1999

Acknowledgements

This book is the product of many contributions: we hope we have done justice to the quality of the 'ingredients' we worked with. Thanks are due, first, to the many project participants, individuals and organizations, who have generously shared their experiences, learning, hopes and fears with us.

That the Relational Health Care project was started and continues is due in no small measure to the support of many committed individuals. We would particularly like to acknowledge the support of Duncan Vere, John Buckler, Eunice Burton, Janet Goodall and John Philpott-Howard, as well as the members of our Advisory Board who have been generous with their time and advice. We are also grateful for the time and freedom to pursue this project provided by the directors of our respective organizations, Valerie Iles and Michael Schluter.

Many people have contributed to our understanding of relationships and methods of assessing them. Particular thanks are due to Mark Scholefield at the Relationships Foundation and Tony Powell at KPMG for their contribution to developing the tools used in the course of the project.

The Health Education Authority commissioned one of the pieces of work which has formed a major part of this project: we are grateful for their permission to reproduce much of the material from the project. We would also like to acknowledge the financial support of Merck, Sharpe and Dohme which has aided the writing of this book.

Finally thanks are due to Susan Sweeney for all her work with the manuscript.

The Relationships Foundation

The Relationships Foundation is a registered charity (No. 327610) established in 1993 and based in Cambridge. Its work is based on the belief that relationships are crucial to the well-being of individuals, families, communities and society as a whole and that they are affected by decisions and actions at all levels – from individuals to neighbourhoods and organizations through to public policy.

The Foundation seeks to promote an agenda for social change that puts a concern for relationships at the heart of public and private life. This involves research projects and practical initiatives to support the development of relationships within and between public sector organizations to improve service delivery, as well as a range of initiatives to support family and community relationships.

The Foundation's current main areas of work include:

- Relational Health Care
- Relational Justice – looking mainly at relationships within the criminal justice system
- Citylife – an Industrial and Provident Society set up by the Foundation to develop city based responses to long-term unemployment
- Relational Business where the Foundation is working in partnership with KPMG
- An international project supporting peace building and reconciliation in Rwanda and Sudan.

For more information on the Relationships Foundation please contact:

Benedicte Scholefield
The Relationships Foundation
Jubilee House
3 Hooper Street
Cambridge
CB1 2NZ

Tel: 01223 566333
Fax: 01223 566359
Email: r.f@clara.net
Web: www.r.f.clara.net

*'Meaningless! Meaningless!
says the Teacher.
Everything is meaningless!'*

*'Not only was the Teacher wise, but also he imparted
knowledge to the people.'*
(Ecclesiastes 12: 8–9)

List of Abbreviations

A and E	Accident and Emergency
BMA	British Medical Association
CHD	Coronary Heart Disease
CHI	Commission for Health Improvement
CHS	Community Health Services
CSR	Comprehensive Spending Review
DHA	District Health Authority
DoH	Department of Health
DPH	Director of Public Health
EL	Executive Letter
FHSA	Family Health Services Authority
GMS	General Medical Services
GPC	General Practice Committee
GPFH	General Practice Fundholder
GP	General Practitioner
HA	Health Authority
HCHS	Hospital and Community Health Services
HEA	Health Education Authority
HIP	Health Improvement Programme
HNA	Health Needs Assessment
HSC	Health Service Circular
HSJ	Health Service Journal
IMT	Information Management and Technology
IPPR	Institute of Public Policy Research
IT	Information Technology
LAC	Local Authority Circular
LHG	Local Health Group
LMC	Local Medical Committee
MDS	Minimum Data Set
NHS	National Health Service
NHSE	National Health Service Executive
NICE	National Institute for Clinical Excellence
ONS	Office of National Statistics
PCAP	Primary Care Act Pilot
PCG	Primary Care Group

List of Abbreviations

PES	Public Expenditure Survey
PGE	Post Graduate Education
PHCT	Primary Health Care Team
PCT	Primary Care Trust
PFI	Private Finance Initiative
PMS	Personal Medical Services
RCGP	Royal College of General Practitioners
RF	Relationships Foundation
RHA	Regional Health Authority
RHC	Relational Health Care
RSM	Royal Society of Medicine
SLA	Service Level Agreement
SSD	Social Services Directorate
TPP	Total Purchasing Pilot
UK	United Kingdom
VFM	Value for Money
WHO	World Health Organisation

1
Agenda

'Since no man knows the future,
who can tell him what is to come?'
(Ecclesiastes 8: 7)

Terms of reference

This is a book for a good day. On a good day the concept of relationship impresses as profound and there is a reasonable chance that the practice may at least aspire to the ideal. On a good day relationships are fundamental. Both the abstract idea and the practical experience satisfy, even to the point of personal fulfilment. This is 'meaning of life' stuff: relationships are at the heart of the matter.

But this is also a book which is needed and designed for a bad day. On a bad day the self-evident efficacy of relationships is disarmingly elusive. The concept itself seems superficial. At worst, in a world of apparently escalating pressures and overwhelming events, change in all its various forms makes the experience of relationships disposable. Their importance becomes transient, peripheral to both policy making and professional practice. The apparent impossibility of attaining meaningful relationships in modern life depresses and demoralizes. This is the backdrop to 'doomsday' scenarios: relationships belong to the notion of a previous 'golden age'.

The contemporary NHS has had its full share of bad days. When four years ago we began the Relational Health Care (RHC) project on which this book is based, we were continuously struck by the despair and, not infrequently, sense of hopelessness which pervaded the outlooks of so many of the healthcare professionals and managers we encountered. These feelings went well beyond concerns about the introduction and implementation of 'internal market' mechanisms in the NHS. Indeed, we met many who applauded the improved levels of performance in terms of, for example, hospital treatment and throughput that the use of purchasing and contracting mechanisms were seen to have brought. The negative feelings were associated rather with the sense that healthcare was becoming a commodity, patients were becoming consumers and that within healthcare organizations the personal and social consequences of organizational developments and decision making were simply not being taken into account.

The consequence was alienation. One NHS chair who was sympathetic to RHC at its inception spoke of the whole NHS labour force – staff and subcontractors alike – 'becoming like a million negative ambassadors'. In 1995/96 it seemed as if every time you met somebody from the NHS at a social function you had to listen to a bad news story: not so much of lengthy waiting lists, but of professional uncertainty, insecure roles and mounting short-term responsibilities.

One simple case example vividly illustrates this condition. In 1995 one of the health authority management teams that was first linked to the project had six members. The oldest was just 43. All bar one had suffered family breakdowns in the previous three years and each one attributed these in large part to the changing state of the NHS and its displaced pressures. This management team was responsible for services with an annual expenditure of more than a billion pounds.

Relationships are important for health and healthcare

The need for the healthcare system in the UK to rediscover the concept and practice of relationships was, in these circumstances, not difficult to assert. Accordingly, the RHC project agenda has been simple and constant. Relationships contribute to health. More than that, relationships actually redefine what is meant by health. This understanding of health has to begin with those working for the organizations charged, in their different ways, with being responsible for delivering better health and healthcare, principally through the NHS. If it does not start here then startlingly the contemporary NHS can at times become self-defeating: creating through its clinical labels more illness and disability; perversely encouraging more referrals and delays by dint of its extra activity-based economic incentives, and maintaining dependence for many patients and much of the public through the preservation of its professional pecking orders. For the NHS the relational perspective was of paramount importance. It offered in 1995/96 a very different way of interpreting such litmus test NHS values as efficiency, effectiveness and equity.

This remains as true today as we reach the year 2000. The political context is very different, of course. As you will read in Chapter 2 ministerial presentations now have an explicitly sympathetic pitch. In terms of policy the relational perspective may well never have it so good again. But the expressed practice and espoused policy may be quite different. In some parts of the 'millennium' NHS, as the case examples in this book often highlight, intention and implementation can often be distant relations. The agenda for RHC has not changed: relationships for health on the one hand and a health system that genuinely stands for relationships on the other.

Target audience

Healthcare professionals are leaders

This is a book for a wide readership. It is also a book for the leadership of the healthcare system. These two targets do not, as they might first appear, face in opposite directions. Decentralization has been a consistent political motif in the NHS over the past decade, regardless of changes in central government. Primary care trusts (PCTs) may now be the prototype, rather than general practice fundholders, but the direction of travel remains firmly towards local resource management, whatever the chosen vehicle for delivery. With this decentralization of operational responsibilities comes the opportunity to influence. The policy community is infinitely broader than it was 10 years ago. There are many more representative organizations at national level. Health-sector journals, books and magazines have proliferated. Above all, the bringing together into a direct encounter of the local and central interfaces – with the public and politicians respectively – of the NHS has created abundant and unprecedented scope for individual initiatives to flourish and take root, not simply in their own patch but elsewhere. This has been a time of transferable learning, when local invention can genuinely be replicated as national innovation.

A few obvious examples of such practical plagiarism illustrate the point. The national NHS Direct Helpline of the year 2000 traces its origins to nurse-led general practice-based telephone advice services such as that set up in Salisbury in 1996 (SWOOP 1997). The Prime Minister's 10-year programme for improved cancer facilities explicitly translates the practice of specialists in Manchester and Glasgow onto the national stage. The rapid creation of such new frontline services as drop-in centres and area-based GP out-of-hours rotas owe their speed of development to the need to catch up centrally, in terms of policy statements and statutory regulations, with mould-breaking entrepreneurial ventures between professionals in individual suburbs and market towns (Hadley and Gordon 1996). Out-of-hours services, for example, were initiated by the GP cooperatives in Bridgewater and the Medway towns; and the PCT concept itself can be traced back directly to the vision of an individual GP setting out his stall at a local surgery in Burnham-on-Crouch (Starey 1996).

In short, while clearly since the 1997 general election there has been a reassertion of central accountabilities – through, for example, the new public service agreements – the process of policy formulation and delivery has become more pluralistic than was ever the case during the first 40 years of the welfare state (Meads 1997a p8–10, Exworthy and Halford 1999). It is now the responsibility and expectation of all health-care professionals to contribute to leadership. The mechanisms are increasingly in place to provide the scope for this to happen. If before 1997 opportunism was the hallmark of effective leadership in terms of making a difference either to policy or practice, such mechanisms as health action zones, primary care groups (PCGs) and above all health improvement programmes (HImPs) appear to offer a new systematic capacity to contribute. HImPs, for example, should be regarded as the first viable framework for the two-way commissioning of health services between professionals in primary and secondary care through, for example, integrated care pathways; as well as a means of extending public participation in the future setting of priorities for health-care investment (and disinvestment).

What has been termed the 'new managerialism' for professionals in healthcare means that the professional role itself is fundamentally changing (Exworthy and Halford 1999, pp1–17). It no longer denotes simply specialist skills and knowledge. By definition now the professional role is inter-professional. Integral to its expression is the responsibility to relate positively to policy and practice development: to contribute as a personal obligation to the way healthcare is planned, organized and reviewed; not just delivered.

With this mindset the book is targeted first and foremost at the care professionals and clinical practitioners at the forefront of this paradigm shift. Accordingly, it is written with clinical directors, nurse practitioners, senior physiotherapists, health managers and their like principally in mind. It is also written with one eye on those who at national and supradistrict level now have the main responsibilities for articulating the organizational and systems developments in the form of the policy guidance and legislation that still shape the overall framework of relationships in healthcare.

Primary care groups: the relationships challenge

The other eye is on PCGs: their members, associates and partners. In the period on which this book is based, 1995–99, the arrival of PCGs was the single most significant change in the NHS. Politically, they symbolized its 'modernization' (Secretary of State for Health 1997, pp32–41). In practical terms they signified a fundamental about-turn in resource control. Before their arrival, 80% of local NHS funds were controlled by hospitals and other NHS provider trusts; only 20% were directly in the gift of GPs and other primary care professionals. Now there is a real prospect of these income proportions being completely reversed. Once converted into NHS trusts, PCGs will become the pivotal units of NHS performance in their local areas.

This change has represented a major relationships challenge. It flies in the face of the history of primary care in the UK. Partnership has always meant between GPs (or dentists) only, not other professionals. Indeed this form of uniprofessional arrangement has been synonymous with general practice since 1948. With PCGs, on paper at least, this changes. Social workers – the old enemy – nurses and members of the public sit down with GPs on the PCG board to make collectively and corporately all sorts of decisions. At times it has been hard to know whether to laugh or to cry. PCGs may be regarded either as audacious in the extreme or the height of naïvety, depending on whether it is a good or a bad day.

The real prospect of too many bad days has meant members of over 200 local primary care organizations have taken part in the RHC project. This participation has

---

Table 1.1. New primary care relationships

Pre-1998/99 general practices	Post-1998/99 primary care organizations
Intrapractice	Social services departments
Health authority	Community nursing team
Provider(s), especially district general	Clinical management groups
hospitals	Local councils
	Local media
(3–4)	Key community groups
	National monitors (eg National Institute
	for Clinical Excellence)
	Health authority
	Finance brokers and banks
	Pharmaceutical companies
	IM&T facilities
	NHS Direct
	Other PCGs or PCTs
	National Primary Care Association/Alliance
	(13–14)
Operational	**Strategic**

(based on analysis of 50 local relational profiles prepared by members of individual PCGs in 1998/99)

taken various forms, ranging from a programme of relational audits and facilitated workshops to simply attending a Relationships Foundation-sponsored conference. It does mean that this book has a primary care bias. For those who turn to it just as a toolkit for primary care organizational development there is a lot on offer. Table 1.1, for example, summarizes the relationships challenge for emerging PCGs nationwide. Based on a simple matrix checklist (see Table 7.1) used in different forms by more than 50 emerging PCGs, it illustrates the dramatic change now taking place in the number and profile of primary care relationships.

Before the mid-1990s the unit of the general practice was still sovereign in primary care. It would on average have three key working relationships:

▶ those within the practice itself

▶ those with the health authority (usually through the residual functions of the family practitioner committee/family health services authority)

▶ those with the main local secondary care provider – usually the district general hospital.

The NHS community health services trust was not normally recognized as a significant separate entity. Its district nurses, health visitors and therapists were seen rather in relation to the practice itself; either within or attached to the primary healthcare team (PHCT).

From 1999/2000 onwards all this changes. The number of key relationships rises from three (or four) to 13 (or 14) for the emerging still GP-led primary care organizations. Their order of importance too is turned on its head. In local workshops participants completing their new relational profiles can often enter into heated discussions over which, for example, is the tenth or twelfth most important 'new partnership'. Health authorities are fortunate now if they appear in the first six of a list prepared by a prospective PCT – with potentially devastating consequences for local ownership of the HImPs. Several new relationships are identified, particularly with commercial and voluntary sector organizations. The single biggest change is in the status afforded social services departments. At a stroke the fallacy of the traditional NHS is exposed. The natural first relationship of general practice is with social not secondary care. The common legacy of a medical education is actually less important in reality than the operational demands for GPs and social workers of being together on the frontline in the community. Indeed, together and with time they may redefine what the public understanding and definition of 'primary care' is.

At this stage, of course, the scale of such changes in relational profiles and their implications leaves the participants feeling ambivalent. Denial mixes with excitement. In force-field analysis terms, there are at least as many stubborn 'mules' waiting to obstruct 'progress' by any means at their disposal, as there are aggressive 'lions' ready to act as new primary care product champions (Lewin 1951). The meanings of such political concepts and values as partnership, (strategic) coordination and integration (Secretary of State for Health 1997, pp10–16) are as yet as ambiguous as the feelings of health professionals are ambivalent. This book is designed to help the participants in contemporary primary care developments and others reach some kind of personal resolution to these dilemmas. It is for each of the specific parts of the healthcare system listed in Table 1.1. But in the last analysis, it has a much more general purpose. The target of the book is those concerned about the condition of the new NHS, especially those concerned to do something to put right its relationships in the interests of health.

Approach

The research framework for this book is action research. Its principal fieldwork methodology is that of participant observation. The basic assumptions underpinning the action research cycle (Fig. 1.1) is that the subject matter for study is inherently and constantly dynamic. To understand the change process requires the engagement of its participants at all stages:

▶ setting of the research objectives

▶ their evaluation and review

▶ subsequent revisions.

The research design in this type of qualitative enquiry must therefore remain ultimately flexible (Bouma and Atkinson 1995). Its techniques have to adapt to the changing behaviour of the project's participants. The perceptions of the latter, rather than a specific set of hypotheses, determine the research questions or issues under examination.

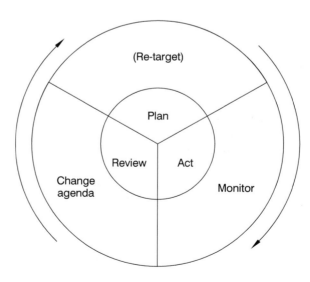

Figure 1.1 Action Research Model (developed from A Edwards and R Talbot (1994).

A community-based descriptive study

Given the selective nature of the evidence, the results of this type of exploratory research are most legitimately considered to be new insights into problems and well-defined priorities for future study, rather than laboratory-standard scientific conclusions (Scott 1965, pp267–71). In the simplest of terms, the RHC project so far has been a community-based descriptive study in which we have taken (some of) the changing relationships of the contemporary NHS (and its associates) as our subject matter, and sought to portray and define its characteristics (Scott 1965) in order to 'generate hypotheses for the solution of a problem' (Muir Gray 1997).

The classic definition of the kind of field work was provided almost 40 years ago in a textbook on social sciences research methodologies published when these were still very much in their infancy:

> *'Fieldwork refers to observations of people in situ; finding them where they are, staying with them in some role which, while acceptable to them, will allow both intimate observations of certain parts of their behaviour, and reporting it in ways useful to social science and not harmful to those observed.'*

(Hughes 1960)

This captures the essence of the RHC approach, except that our aspiration has been to move beyond being 'not harmful' to reporting in ways which are actually helpful. This has largely been through the mechanism of the local workshops, mostly involving PCGs, which constitute the majority of the settings for 'observations of people *in situ*'. These workshops were not dependent on the RHC project for their instigation. They were rather part of the organizational development processes of the contemporary NHS and its associates, to which we were attached and in which we then participated as facilitators, reviewers or *raporteurs*.

These opportunities for participant observation, each explicitly negotiated, required an acute awareness of the fundamental difficulties arising from this approach. As Whyte (1943) emphasized in his pioneering study of delinquency and deviance well before the time of the classic statement by Hughes on fieldwork above, there is the constant danger of becoming a non-participating observer on the one hand and on the other, of falling into the trap of becoming a non-observing participant as social situations and identities change. To be conscious of these perils and developments requires personal and professional discipline, augmented in our case by the expert oversight of the project's advisory board, details of which are given in Appendix A. Its regular scrutiny and feedback has been important in retaining focus, setting future directions and, above all, helping to give relevant meanings to events. It represented a significant element in what one social scientist described as the need for participant observers to subject themselves to a continuous 'process of self-objectification' (Vidich 1954).

Participant observation through local workshops and audits, augmented by supplementary material from RHC conferences and focus groups, constituted the 'act' (and monitor) stage in the action research cycle (Fig. 1.1). The work of the focus groups on 'competition', 'collaboration' and 'caring' supplied much of the raw material for Chapters 3, 6 and 7. This book clearly represents the third and final stage in the initial research cycle: the 'review' designed to reflect and identify the change agenda. Its findings are summarized in terms of 'prospects' for the new NHS in Chapter 10.

There was, of course, also the initial planning stage, which comprises a full third of Edwards and Talbot's research model (1994, p10). It is in this first stage that the targets are set and reset. It is time to take aim.

Aims

The seven objectives of the RHC project are listed in Table 1.2, as redefined in May 1999. These updated those set in October 1996 and which had included the RHC target of a relational perspective in national policy statements and conference agendas by 1998. Clearly, in 1999 this was neither necessary nor applicable. The focus had shifted from communicating the concepts and principles to converting them into practice.

A substantial amount of intelligence gathering and information analysis took place at the initial planning stage between September 1995 and September 1997. This had a twin focus. The first was on health itself. With financial support from such sympathetic sponsors as the Jubilee Centre and the Bible Society, an extensive literature review was undertaken to identify the different models of health and their relational components. From this a detailed analysis was prepared (and published) of the empirical evidence associating changes in relationships and social support to specific impacts on the human immune system, thereby linking individual disease and illness patterns to such causal factors as stress, negative life events and relational dysfunction (Susans C, personal communication 1997, Jubilee Centre 1998).

The second focus was on gaining a better understanding of NHS relationships themselves. With support from the King's Fund and Churchill Livingstone, research papers were produced (and published) that critically appraised the impacts of central policy and organizational developments on such significant NHS interfaces as those with social services departments and community health services trusts (Robson 1997, Lewis 1997). A full list of RHC publications and papers is contained in Appendix B.

From this early investigative work it was clear that the deep concerns which led to the inception of the RHC project were being borne out. Virtually all the traditional relationships upon which the very viability of the NHS depended were under threat:

▶ doctor and patient

▶ national institution and citizen

▶ demarcation of public and private sector boundaries

▶ above all, healthcare professionals with general management.

The fears of those who asked the Relationships Foundation to start the RHC initiative in 1995/96 – several of whom were of high standing in the NHS – were broadly confirmed. By the end of the project's planning stage it had 300 subscribing supporters who saw in such recurring crises as rising waiting lists, escalating

Table 1.2. Relational healthcare: the targets

Overall aim: To help ensure that the relational concept takes root in both national policy developments for health and the local practice of healthcare

Specific objectives:

▶ Further development of a network of people at the grass roots committed to RHC through the distribution of regular communications on relational best practice in different parts of the healthcare system
▶ Inclusion of proven relational assessment methodologies within NHS performance management and regulation arrangements
▶ Critical analysis and constructive appraisal of central policies from a relational perspective in ways that exert effective influence
▶ Application of relational audit and development programmes to local situations where participants are willing to share learning nationally, at a rate of at least three per annum
▶ Consultancy as required, by the Relationships Foundation or on its behalf, with those parts of the changing health system where relationship needs are most pronounced
▶ Active support of up to 20 identified national healthcare leaders prepared to promote RHC
▶ Production of regular publications on RHC which ensure a national interest

(October 1996, updated May 1999)

prescribing costs, ward closures and mental illness breakdowns not so much the economic costs and political consequences as the absence of the relationships required, if not for solutions, then at least for something that might be regarded as an appropriate remedy or palliative.

Table 1.3 details the components of this initial planning stage within the framework of the action research cycle (Fig. 1.1). It led to the decision to target for action in the second stage, between October 1997 and July 1999, the monitoring of the most prominent and profound organizational changes taking place in the health system. These were those of primary care in the first instance; and health authorities in the second as they underwent major reductions in size and number, and had to make the profound changes in substance, systems and style that moving from the operational responsibilities of purchasing to the strategic responsibilities of regulation and overall performance management require.

During this second stage RHC project members undertook workshops, audits and allied interventions with primary care organizations and other healthcare agencies in England, Scotland and Wales. With financial support from such bodies as the Health Education Authority and a number of individual health authorities and NHS trusts, these opportunities for participant observation concentrated on three areas:

▶ inter-professional team development

▶ health strategy formulation

▶ interorganizational collaboration.

Again this part of the research programme has led to a number of publications (Bemain 1999; Meads *et al* 1999; Meads 1999).

This book represents a large part of the final review stage in this action research cycle. It is structured deliberately around the generic constituents of any (health) system: policy, resources, strategy, organization, delivery, development, review and

Table 1.3. Research schedule

Stage	Dates
A Planning	
Establishment of project advisory board	June 1995
Literature and documentation reviews and selected interviews in NHS	June to Sept 1995
Three seminars in Leeds, London and Oxford to listen to concerns about relationships in health from a broad cross-section of health professionals and managers	Autumn 1995
Preparation of reports on condition of NHS relationships and contribution of relationships to variable health status	Aug 1995 to Feb 1997
Terms of reference and RHC objectives drafted and agreed, with action plan	Oct 1996
Early publications (Robson 1996, Susans 1997) and first RHC newsletter issued	From summer 1996
B Action	
Relational audit with a health authority and NHS community trust in London successfully piloted	March to July 1997
Workshop programme with health care organizations commences	Sept 1997
Partnership HEA programme to evaluate relationship between new primary care organizations and public health, with six relational profiling exercises and workshops undertaken	From Jan 1998
Facilitation of 50 plus newly formed PCGs using RHC development material	From April 1998
Cambridge based training courses for PCG consultants and managers	Sept 1998 and April 1999
Quarterly advisory board meetings	Ongoing
Series of update articles published in relevant healthcare journals (Lewis 1997, Meads 1997b, 1998, 1999, Bemain 1999)	Oct 1997 to March 1999 1997–98
Contributions to 'New NHS' national conferences by RHC project members	Ongoing
C Review	
Advisory board membership reviewed and extended (eg to include non-NHS organizations)	Oct 1998
Book contracts and funding secured with HEA/RSM/MSD to ensure publication of project findings	Dec 1998
Original project objectives updated and revised	May 1999
First RHC book published	June 1999
Future change agenda for both new NHS and RHC project addressed in Relational Foundation Corporate Strategy	July 1999
Relationships in the NHS delivered to publisher	Aug 1999

quality. While inevitably much of the case material deployed in the forthcoming chapters is topical and transitory, the themes are not. They belong to all systems: hence the selection of chapter headings. The final one, Chapter 10, is 'Prospects'. In this we revisit our original remit as participant observers to offer new insights into new situations and the problems they bring with them; and to suggest and define the priorities for future research-based practice and policy.

It is the subject of policy to which we turn first in Chapter 2. In this the style and sequence of the book are set: a selective analysis of contemporary policy followed by a constructive appraisal of how RHC can contribute. In considering this axis, a series of practical aids are suggested, drawn from the action stage of the research cycle. The aim is to bridge the gap between intention and implementation. Never before in the life cycle of the NHS has such assistance been so needed.

Summary

The RHC project has its origins in a widespread disillusionment about the state of relationships in the NHS and their impact on health. Over the period 1995–99 it has followed an action research model with new primary care organizations offering abundant opportunities for participant observation. The lessons of RHC are applicable, however, across the whole UK health system.

References

Bouma GD and Atkinson GB (1995). *A Handbook of Social Science Research*. Oxford: Oxford University Press: 210.
Bemain R (1999). Front line workers. *British Journal of Health Care Management* **5** (Suppl): 2–5.
Edwards A and Talbot R (1994). *The Hard-Pressed Researcher*. London: Longman.
Exworthy M and Halford S, eds (1999). *Professionals and the New Managerialism in the New Public Sector*. Buckingham: Open University Press.
Hadley J and Gordon P, eds (1996). *Extending Primary Care*. Oxford: Radcliffe Medical Press.
Hughes EC (1960). The place of field work in social science. In: Junker BF, ed. *Fieldwork: An Introduction to the Social Sciences*. Chicago: University of Chicago Press: v–xv.
Jubilee Centre (1998). *Biblical Perspectives on Health and Health Care*. Cambridge: Jubilee Centre.
Lewin K (1951). *Field Theory in Social Sciences*. New York: Harper and Row.
Lewis C (1997). Enhancing collaboration in primary care. *Primary Care* **7**(10): 5–6.
Meads G (1997a). *Power and Influence in the NHS*. Oxford: Radcliffe Medical Press: 8–10.
Meads G (1997b). The relational challenge. *Health Management* **9**: 22–3.
Meads G (1998). Integrated primary care: The relational challenge. *Journal of Integrated Care* **2**: 51–4.
Meads G (1999). Research matrix reveals real typology of primary care groups. *British Journal of Health Care Management* **5**(3): 96–100.
Meads G, Killoran A, Ashcroft J, Cornish Y (1999). *Mixing Oil and Water*. London: HEA Publications.
Muir Gray JA (1997). *Evidence-Based Healthcare*. London: Churchill Livingstone: 100.
Robson T (1997). *NHS/Social Services Relationships*. Cambridge: Relationships Foundation.
Scott WR (1965). Field methods in the study of organisations. In: March JG, ed. *Handbook of Organisations*. Chicago: Rand McNally: 261–304.
Secretary of State for Health (1997). *The New NHS: Modern, Dependable*, Cm 3807. London: HMSO.
Starey N (1996). The primary care trust: Co-ordination for cohesion. In: Meads G, ed. *Future Options for General Practice*. Oxford: Radcliffe Medical Press: 165–89.
SWOOP (South Wiltshire Out Of Hours Project) (1997). Nurse telephone triage in out-of-hours primary care: a pilot study. *British Medical Journal* **314**: 198–9.
Vidich AJ (1954). Participant observation and the collection and interpretation of data. *American Journal of Sociology* **60**: 345–60.
Whyte WF (1943). *Street Corner Society*. Chicago: University of Chicago Press: 357.

2
Policy

'The more the words,
the less the meaning . . . '
(Ecclesiastes 6: 11)

Stated agenda

The importance of policy needs no telling in a public service which has been so significantly shaped and reshaped over the past decade by policies introducing an internal
market, pointing the way to a primary care-led NHS and seeking a healthier nation. Yet
for all its impact, and indeed the improvements in healthcare that good policies wisely
implemented can bring, many health professionals are still tempted to regard policy as
unimportant: something for others who have the inclination; likely to be a departure
from clinical common-sense; and an unwelcome intrusion into the daily business of
providing healthcare. After so much recent rapid change there is an understandable
weariness and wariness.

This chapter is not designed as a comprehensive analysis of contemporary health
policy. Rather, it is an account of how the many parts of the NHS with which we have
worked have engaged with policy, and the implications of this involvement for the
development of more relational healthcare. Many of the details of policy are picked up
in subsequent chapters in so far as they affect the core functions of the health service.
Here, therefore, we are more concerned with people's experience of the process of
policy making and implementation.

Policy can be expected to divide an ambivalent service: between the cynics and
sceptics and the enthusiasts and visionaries; between the mules (resisting change) and
the lions (champions for change) (Lewin 1951); as well as between competing health
ideologies, professional interests and pressure groups. These divisions, just as much as
different forms of unity, pervade issues and relationships. The important issues at stake
include achieving the integration of care, which has been long discussed but rarely
achieved; and seeing real improvements in the quality of care and public health. There
are also many relationships at stake: policy shapes the relationship between the individual patient and health professional and between communities and their local health
systems; and provides the external accountabilities for the medical professions in their
relationships with the public. Policy making and implementation depend upon the
relationships between government departments to achieve real 'joined-up' government
(Dobson F, speech to NHS Confederation Annual Conference, 25 June 1997), as well
as between policy makers and service providers to ensure that policy results in the
delivery of desired outcomes. Policy shapes the relationships within the health system

through the structures it creates, as well as through authorizing such processes as commissioning or performance management. Policy may also act as an arbiter of competing interests regarding, for example, resource allocation or influence.

Modernizing the NHS

Current Department of Health policy is influenced by a number of broader policy themes, most notably modernization and devolution, although it is of course formulated within Treasury-set parameters. Modern policy and public service will, according to the white paper *Modernising Government* (Minister for the Cabinet Office 1999) be:

▶ *Pragmatic*: in 'third way' politics 'what counts is what works'. The intention is that 'freed from the dogmas that haunted governments of the past', modern policy should be free to find new and better ways of delivering the services people want. The retention of the Private Finance Initiatives (PFIs) is cited as an example of this policy which eschews a doctrinaire approach.

▶ *Inclusive*: this applies both to the process of policy making and provision of services. Leading the debate on how to improve policy means 'developing new relationships between Whitehall, the devolved administrations [in Scotland, Wales and Northern Ireland], local government and the voluntary and private sectors; consulting outside experts, those who implement policy and those affected by it early in the policy making process' (Minister for the Cabinet Office 1999, p16). In service provision, inclusiveness means providing equitably for all people and making contributions which tackle social exclusion. This requires flexibility as 'there is no such thing as a typical citizen as people's needs and concerns differ: between men and women, for example; between the young and old, and between people of different social, cultural and educational backgrounds; and people with disabilities' (Minister for the Cabinet Office, 1.16). For the NHS this has meant a greater focus on public health, tackling health inequalities and the abolition of such allegedly inequitable two-tier systems as fundholding.

▶ *Integrated*: 'policies and programmes, local and national, tackle the issues facing society – like crime, drugs, housing and environment – in a joined up way, regardless of the organizational structure of government' (Minister for the Cabinet Office 1999, 1.7). For the NHS this has meant a particular emphasis on collaboration and the 'duty of partnership' so that all parts of the health system work together to provide seamless care for the whole person and the whole community. The concern for integration is broad-based and includes, for example, the relationships between the NHS, local authorities and voluntary agencies in pursuing public health.

▶ *Committed to quality*: 'we will deliver efficient, high quality public services and will not tolerate mediocrity' (Minister for the Cabinet Office, Ch 4). This is a twin-track policy. Modern government is intended to foster innovation, creativity and skills in improving services. This is designed to be coupled with tough performance management, bringing people up to the standards of the best and making the best better. Clear targets are to be set through public service agreements, including reductions in waiting lists, with performance management shifting towards outcome measures. New central bodies such as the National Institute for Clinical Excellence (NICE) are being set up to help ensure improved quality standards across the country.

► *'Information-age'*: 'we will use new technology to meet the needs of citizens and not trail behind technological developments' (Minister for the Cabinet Office, Ch 5). The emphasis is on accessibility and efficiency. Technology is seen as offering new ways of accessing services and information at times and places which may be more convenient to the user. Efficiency is to be enhanced through better information management. For the NHS this has meant the rapid roll-out of NHS Direct – a direct telephone link for nursing advice – as well as other initiatives such as the NHSnet.

► *Long-term*: modern policy is intended to be forward-looking, moving beyond short-term reactive policy making to engage fully with the root causes of issues and not just their symptoms. This is important for issues such as social exclusion and public health where significant progress has to be a long-term prospect. It is still, of course, open to question how consistently a long-term agenda will be allowed to shape day-to-day delivery and policy implementation.

A modern NHS sounds good, although its aspirations are not new. Quality, equity, integration and inclusiveness have always been important values, at least in parts of the NHS. The challenge of modernization, if it is to have any bite, lies in the cultural changes that it implies and this is where the tensions and disagreements may be expected to arise. Modernization talks of 'unlocking the potential' of 'effective partnerships for improving public health' (NHS Executive 1998a, 1998b). But potential can all too easily be constrained again by new structures and inappropriate performance management. Trying to effect cultural change can be destabilizing and risky, and ambitious targets are hard to reach. Policy can often presume a higher starting base than in fact exists. As the following chapters will show, bridging the gap between intention and implementation will at times demand more than a considerable leap of faith.

Devolution and decentralization

Devolution has resulted in separate white papers and consultation documents for England (Secretary of State for Health 1997), Scotland (Secretary of State for Scotland 1997), Wales (Secretary of State for Wales 1998) and Northern Ireland (Department of Health and Social Services 1998). These set out the changes to the UK health system which potentially make it more capable of delivering the government's health agenda (although what the real agenda is, and the extent to which health systems will be capable of delivering it, is not yet entirely clear).

The intention is that overall policy is integrated so that people in, for example, Portsmouth, Perth and Pembroke can expect broadly similar healthcare. There are indeed strong common themes such as the determination to restore an NHS based on partnership and collaboration and to uphold the basic principles of a universally available NHS, free at the point of need and funded through general taxation. But there are also significant differences which reflect local contexts and may give rise to health systems with differing capabilities. Only in England will NHS community trusts remain, at least for now, although for most areas they are likely to form part of primary care trusts (PCTs) where their links to the community and public health capacity will be an important resource. In Scotland there is no framework for the primary care commissioning of secondary care. In Wales the relationship between the people and the newly elected National Assembly in Cardiff starts to take precedence in policy statements over the relationship between the individual and professional.

Devolution of power is not applied consistently in the different white papers. In England we are seeing a significant shift of financial control to primary care groups (PCGs). The political significance of this should not pass unnoticed; after many years of seeing power increasingly centralized, the possibility of NHS PCTs becoming genuine community healthcare organizations, with a high degree of public ownership and involvement and controlling some 80% of NHS spending, could mark a significant shift of power back to localities.

An uncertain agenda

We have encountered real uncertainty and ambivalence within (and outside) the NHS in response to current health policies. This has been about:

- ▶ what the real health agenda is

- ▶ the balance between long-term goals and the political pressures for successful initiatives in the short term

- ▶ the balance between local and central control in implementing policy

- ▶ the openness of government in developing policy

- ▶ the impact of policy on key healthcare relationships, in particular those between GP and patient and between the different professions themselves

- ▶ above all, perhaps, whether current policy is in the end essentially about further structural change (with a focus on quality, accountability and cost control), or whether it is seeking the stated changes in culture and behaviour to achieve integrated care and improved public health.

In our work with many districts and provider organizations to support policy implementation, we have often found considerable uncertainty as to what the real policy agenda is. This arises from cynicism about the real motives, widely perceived 'initiativitis' – which can make it hard to discern the policy vision behind the plethora of initiatives – and mixed messages from performance management exercised at central and regional levels. Thus, for some people health improvement programmes (HImPs) are the heart of the policy agenda, while others see them merely as the 'n'th initiative in the pile, to be pursued after others, such as waiting list targets, which are perceived to have much tougher and more immediate accountability mechanisms. This has been evident in the very different practical responses. One district health authority management team that we visited deferred the HImP for a year and rebadged the existing purchasing plans, whereas others have invested considerable time in a broadly-based stakeholder consultation process. How time is invested is a good indicator of perceived priorities and the real policy agenda, whether by design or default, will be where accountability and performance management are most stringent. This does not and inevitably will not always match the logical priorities or the vision of central policy statements. We have found that the lack of convergence is often most apparent in local primary care settings.

A public health agenda?

It is certainly possible to see public health at the heart of policy, bringing together the concern for inclusiveness (through tackling health inequalities), integration (through its emphasis on multi-agency collaborative working around HImPs) and quality, supported by reforms to primary care to create a renewed ('modern') health system capable of delivering the policy. Public health, however, has not always been at the heart of recent health policy developments. Primary care, by contrast, has been under the spotlight for several years, at times quite intensively with, for example, no fewer than four major governmental policy initiatives within the space of nine months in 1996/7. These were designed both to extend and reinforce the role of the GP as the managing agent for secondary services and the principal focus for healthcare [(NHS Executive 1996a,b,c) which together led to the 1997 NHS (Primary Care) Act]. Much of the policy has been concerned with the management of medical care, although it is possible to chart a direction of travel from primary medical care to primary managed care (with overall responsibilities for commissioning), through to population-based primary healthcare (Table 2.1). Whether or when this last step will be fully taken is not yet certain.

More recent policy, however, considered overall does have a strong public health focus. According to the July 1999 White Paper *Saving Lives: Our Healthier Nation*, primary care has been placed 'at the heart of our programme to modernize the health service' (Secretary of State for Health 1999). New primary care organizations (PCGs and, in the future, NHS PCTs) are seen as consisting of broadly-based multiprofessional teams for whom 'improving the health of, and addressing inequality in, the local community' is a primary function. A broad socio-economic model of health is also adopted. So, for example, the *Independent Inquiry into Inequalities in Health* acknowledged the influence of a complex mix of factors on health:

> 'Individual lifestyles are embedded in social and community networks and in living and working conditions, which in turn are related to the wider cultural and socio-economic environment . . . . Socio-economic inequalities in health reflect differential exposure – from before birth and across the lifespan'- to risk associated with socio-economic position.'
>
> (Acheson 1998)

Table 2.1. Primary health care: the direction of travel

	Primary medical care	Primary managed care		Primary health care
Organizational unit	Individual family health services professionals, eg GPs	General practice units	Primary health services	Primary care organizations
Mechanisms for delivery	Via standard national contract	Via business plans, corporate contracts	Via practice contracts	Via long-term local covenants
Service focus	Individual patients	Specified target groups, eg over 75s, under 5s	Practice population	Local communities
Key Transitional Dates	1989	1994	1997	1999

[based on Meads *et al* (1999), p3]

This view of public health has been adopted by the government's public health white paper, *Saving Lives*. The roles and responsibilities of the various parts of the health system are defined in a 'national contract' for health improvement which provides the basis for tackling fragmentation and short termism, two of the main 'enemies' identified. The national contract for health improvement specifies four priority areas: heart disease and stroke, accidents, cancer and mental health. There is an expectation that these will be combined with specific local priorities. This language of contract is also bolstered by the government's new public service agreements which define specific expectations of what services should be provided. Accordingly, HImPs provide the focus for collaborative partnership working to improve the health and wellbeing of communities. The new NHS performance framework reflects this shift of focus with health improvement indicators that monitor variations in health outcomes as well as fairness of access.

The New NHS (Secretary of State for Health 1997) and *Modern Local Government* (Secretary of State for Environment, Transport and the Regions 1998) can be seen as concerned with establishing a health system capable of delivering improved public health, as illustrated in terms of reducing health inequalities and increasing the length of people's lives and the number of years spent free from illness. Local authorities are much more explicitly regarded as an integral part of the health system. Specific initiatives support the implementation of policy: 26 health action zones are being set up to tackle health inequalities and healthy living centres are to be the focus for interagency action for community health at the local level, especially in deprived areas.

The renewed focus on public health, which according to *Saving Lives* is 'reactivating a dormant duty of the NHS', is not intended to consist solely of additional initiatives, but to be evident throughout the NHS. Modernizing the NHS 'is not simply an agenda for improving the reliability and effectiveness of healthcare services. It is an agenda which will help to improve health overall and to tackle inequality. But above all it is PCGs which are expected to 'deliver the agenda'. Their range of public health functions is summarized in Table 2.2.

Promoting public health is not a safe agenda. In a recent project sponsored by the Health Education Authority, in which we looked at how primary care organizations

Table 2.2. Public health functions of PCGs [from Meads *et al* (1999), pp4–5]

- ► Contributing to the development of the local HImP and health action zone plans
- ► Assessing health needs which will be reflected in primary care investment plans and their contribution to the local HImP
- ► Direct responses to community health problems based on collaboration with other organizations and drawing on existing public health and health promotion skills
- ► Securing equitable access to and quality of primary care services for communities through primary care investment plans
- ► Considering use of flexibilities provided by personal medical services pilot projects to develop services that respond in new ways to the health needs of vulnerable groups and deprived communities
- ► Delivering quality standards through new national service frameworks that cover health promotion disease prevention, diagnosis, treatment, rehabilitation and care; with coronary heart disease and mental health representing early frameworks to be applied
- ► Commissioning patient services and managing new developments that are targeted on local health needs, based on evidence of clinical and cost-effectiveness, and produce an optimal balance between primary, community and secondary care services
- ► Providing opportunities for practitioners to work with public health practitioners (health visitors, health promotion specialists, community workers); as well as health authority public health staff and others to undertake needs assessment, interagency work on public health issues, health promotion and disease prevention, and community development work
- ► Being accountable through the annual review process for contributing to health improvement targets

could improve public health as well as deliver healthcare, we found over the 1997–98 period that the organizational types which were most prevalent, or ostensibly most efficient and effective, had the least capacity for public health (see Table 4.3). As these illustrate, it is far from clear whether public health, performance management and clinical governance will actually represent an integrated agenda.

Nor will it be an entirely welcome agenda. Some GPs who have participated in projects have been excited by the opportunities and the vision, but have feared that their colleagues may need to be bought off rather than buy in. Equity will not necessarily be a unifying agenda for a service where the inverse care law of more services and fewer resources often still applies. Incomes and professional influence may be adversely affected. Some remain deeply sceptical that initiatives will translate into tangible benefits. The jury is still out and is unlikely to return a unanimous verdict.

Uncertain relationships

In the early days of the current government administration there appeared to be uncertainty about the style of the relationship: was 'New Labour' really new or would there be a quick reversion to the style of previous Labour administrations? Gaining a feel for the style of the relationship and confidence in its operation has taken time and there are still areas where trust, confidence and understanding need to continue to grow. An important area of uncertainty has been the balance between central control and local freedoms. This applies to such issues as resource allocation where there has been a concern about the appropriate balance between allocation to centrally directed initiatives and to local distribution (and hence greater local responsibility for delivering the agenda), as well as the implementation of key policies such as decentralization through PCGs.

This uncertainty has been evident on all sides. Accordingly, for example, within government there appears to have been initial surprise at the demands for detailed operational guidance on PCG implementation, while for those implementing policy uncertainty has at times resulted in caution and dependency. Working with health authorities to support PCG implementation we found some almost paralysed in the 1998/99 cycle, aware of the scale of the task to be delivered to a tight timetable, yet fearful of running too far ahead of the emerging agenda and delivery guidelines and then having to undo work that is subsequently found not to fit the guidelines.

In extreme cases this proved dispiriting and disempowering where some successful emerging primary care developments, in which much had been invested, were running into the sand as they were feared not to fit well enough with emerging guidance on white paper implementation. Local arrangements for rehabilitation and outpatient clinics are just two examples of this situation that we encountered in Moorgreen and Lambeth. This was emotionally damaging for the participants who then found it difficult fully to commit to implementing new programmes.

Nationally we found wide variations in confidence and approaches to policy implementation. Some parts of the NHS were adept at compliance – ahead of timetable, but at the price of missing the vision and challenge of policy. Some seemed to have the confidence (and the earned licence) to make policy fit their local plans and contexts (eg Dorset), while others were almost reduced to automatons, too intimidated by continual organizational change and fearful for their own personal futures really to take up the challenge and opportunities that the policies present.

Building trust and confidence

An associated problem has been the fear, or perceived lack of tolerance, of failure. A politicized service that will not tolerate mediocrity does not always sit easily with encouragement to experiment and innovate. The dangers of risk aversion are acknowledged:

> *'the culture of parliament, ministers and the civil service create a situation in which the rewards for success are limited and penalties for failure can be severe. The system is too often risk averse.'*
>
> (Minister for the Cabinet Office 1999, 1.11)

Part of the proposed solution is to 'identify organizations which would benefit from being given additional scope to innovate, and consider how to give them appropriate freedoms'. This is a relational issue: reconciling a crusade for quality through innovation on the one hand and tough performance management on the other requires trust and confidence, which must be nurtured and sustained by appropriate systems. Within the NHS this will require changes to the performance management culture to incorporate, on a systematic basis, process measures as part of the modern approach to quality (see Chapter 9).

Policy in the new, modern NHS requires those involved in the development and delivery of policy to learn new working relationships. There is a sense in which health has been politicized with the relationship between government and the public taking precedence over that between patients and service providers. This is most explicit in Wales where primary responsibility for healthcare provision is vested in the Welsh Assembly, with the professional relationships of service provision coming under the aegis of this national contract. It is also evident in England where, for example, manifesto pledges on waiting lists and breast cancer targets make government directly accountable to the public and sections of the national community for aspects of service delivery.

At times this may create an uneasy three-way relationship between government, the NHS and the public. On the one hand there is the need to create distance to strengthen advocacy and accountability, while on the other there is the vision of partnership between government and public services in the common aim of service renewal and improvement. The danger is that those in the NHS are pulled in different directions with service providers becoming closer to the populations they serve, while those shaping policy and regulating performance are drawn closer to government. The risk is recognized in *Modernising Government* as:

> *'an increasing separation between policy and delivery [which] has acted as a barrier to involving in policy making those people who are responsible for delivery on the front line'.*
>
> (Minister for the Cabinet Office 1999)

The opportunity to realign relationships follows from this awareness.

Uncertainty about the balance between local and central influence is also reflected in concerns about openness in the policy process. On the one hand there is considerable openness. Pragmatic evolutionary policy means that today's local initiative can become tomorrow's national programme or beacon site. National conferences, seminars and research and development projects have provided opportunities to take soundings, test ideas and report on progress (and obstacles to progress). The diversity of today's NHS inevitably means there is scope for local innovation and experimentation. The move towards PCGs and eventually NHS PCTs illustrates the evolutionary nature of policy. A direction has been set but neither the precise path nor the final destination is known with any degree of certainty. Many individuals and organizations are helping to chart the way forward and thereby influence policy, with the almost infinite range of community hospital models in England and Wales now a classic example of this development paradigm (Tucker 1999).

Yet on the other hand there remains widespread suspicion of hidden agendas and deals in (nowadays not so) smoke-filled rooms; concerns about the adequacy of consultation and failure to listen to concerns about the speed of change from a tired NHS. One of the persistent lessons from our work has been that whoever you ask in the NHS, power is perceived to lie elsewhere. This is in part a consequence of the many different kinds of power – to allocate resources, to ensure delivery, to influence policy or to obstruct change. Yet it also reflects the increasing size and complexity of the NHS relational map. We have found that everybody's 'rich picture' for the future is different. The multiplication of stakeholders makes power and influence more diffuse and uncertain. There are lessons from past experience here. When inclusiveness results in fragmented or indecisive involvement it can, perversely, lead to less consultation as ineffective processes encourage unilateral decisiveness. Inclusive relationships need careful and diligent management.

Current policy, therefore, if it is to be implemented effectively, depends on building and maintaining the right relationships between those formulating and implementing policy. Despite a surge of optimism when the current political administration entered government, these relationships remain ambiguous and uncertain. Current policy also depends on the relationships which support healthcare delivery. As Chapters 4–6 indicate, there are still parts of the NHS where the relationships will struggle to sustain the appropriate strategic process, organizational developments and delivery of healthcare.

Policy depends on relationships, but also sets out to change them. From a relational perspective, current policy has much to commend it. It seriously engages with the issues arising from the contribution of relationships to health and healthcare. However defined, the health of the nation is not as good as it could or should be. Partnerships that enable integrated whole person care and tackle the causes as well as the symptoms of ill health are welcome.

The ultimate test of current policy will be its impact on patients. Throughout the new NHS there is considerable frustration about not being able to do better for patients. As Chapter 6 shows, current policy provides the opportunity to do this. But is it in the words of one Relational Health Care (RHC) project participant 'a policy too good for the NHS?' Whether the real agenda matches the rhetoric; whether the relationships can sustain the implementation and whether the NHS, with all the legacies of the past, will take the opportunity or find it an unsustainable burden remains to be seen. The first steps will depend on the NHS' resources and the ways in which it perceives and deploys them.

Summary

The new NHS seeks to create a more integrated, modernized service which will improve public health and provide high-quality care through a decentralized healthcare system. The reality does not always match the rhetoric, especially where the NHS remains uncertain about the real agenda and the balance of local and central control; where relationships of trust and confidence between government and NHS have not been created; and where the legacy of previous policies has left people weary and wary. Current policy sets out to change healthcare relationships and the policy process depends upon them. The obstacles to both are considerable.

References

Acheson D (Chair) (1998). *Independent Inquiry into Inequalities in Health*. London: HMSO: 8.
Department of Health and Social Services (1998). *Fit for the Future*. Belfast: Northern Ireland Office.
Lewin K (1951). *Field Theory in Social Sciences*. New York: Harper and Row.
Meads G, Killoran A, Ashcroft J, Cornish Y (1999). *Mixing Oil and Water*. London: Health Education Authority.
Minister for the Cabinet Office (1999). *Modernising Government*, Cm 4310. London: HMSO.
NHS Executive (1996a). *Choice and Opportunity*. London: Department of Health.
NHS Executive (1996b). *Primary Care: The Future*. London: Department of Health.
NHS Executive (1996c). *Delivering the Future*. London: Department of Health.

NHS Executive (1998a). *Better Health and Better Health Care*, HSC 1998/021. London: Department of Health.

NHS Executive (1998b). *Unlocking the Potential*. London: North Thames Regional Office.

Secretary of State for Environment, Transport and the Regions. *Modern Local Government: In Touch with the People*, Cm 4041. London: HMSO.

Secretary of State for Health (1997). *The New NHS: Modern, Dependable*, Cm 3807. London: HMSO.

Secretary of State for Health (1998). *Our Healthier Nation*. London: HMSO.

Secretary of State for Health (1999). *Saving Lives: Our Healthier Nation*. London: HMSO.

Secretary of State for Scotland (1997). *Designed to Care*, Cm 3811. Edinburgh: HMSO.

Secretary of State for Wales (1998). *Putting Patients First*, Cm 3841. Cardiff: HMSO.

Tucker H (1999). *Directory of Community Hospitals*. Bristol: Community Hospitals Association.

3
Resources

'Better one handful with tranquillity,
than two handfuls with toil . . . '
(Ecclesiastes 4: 6)

Relative values

It is tempting to begin and end this chapter with a single sentence. We need to recognize that relationships are our most important resource. In healthcare, as in other walks of life, it is as simple as that.

Relationships are a neglected resource

Or is it? When the NHS issues its official resource assumptions, the currency referred to is not relationships but money. In university settings it is possible to teach health policy perfectly legitimately through the literature and research on public finance. For example, the changing frameworks for capital allocation have clearly been a critical factor in determining the institutional profile of healthcare in the UK; from the standard model district general hospitals of the early 1980s to the closure of long-stay hospitals for patients with mental illnesses and learning difficulties a decade later. The Private Finance Initiative (PFI) today is similarly influential in the physical shaping of such concepts as 'intermediate care' and the ('high-tech') 'hospital without walls'.

The new sophistication in financial audit processes has paved the way for corporate governance and, above all, the whole alignment of clinical and cost-effectiveness has been derived from the health economist's new capacity to quantify the relative financial value (of different surgical procedures and medical interventions) in terms of price-tagged added life quality. In our work with primary care groups, (PCGs) board members in, for example, Lincolnshire, Bridgewater and Camden have prepared their local lists of mid-term priorities, which invariably include comparative costing exercises on both high volume and high price secondary care specialisms – usually under the guise of integrated care pathways – as well, of course, as their own prescribing expenditure at individual practice levels (Table 3.1).

In terms of health policy development it would be inconceivable not to take into account the financial consequences of change. The political and professional implications are similarly a prerequisite for consideration. Through such bodies as the National Institute for Clinical Excellence (NICE) there is now a sharper focus on the consequences of new policies in terms of clinical efficacy. But still the relational perspective is sidelined. Moving the money around without really thinking through what this means remains a singularly British characteristic. In much of Europe and the

Table 3.1. PCG resource management – local example (based on Somerset Coast PCG Development Workshop, June 1999)

Must do's (1999/2000)
► Establish baseline of clinical activity (including hospital episodes and referrals, and individual practice's service activity profiles) with comparative cost analysis

Will do's (2000/2001)
► Develop relevant IM&T
► External communications strategy
► Health needs assessment

Would like to do (2001/2002)
► Define and deliver integrated care pathways – specifically for prostate conditions, coronary heart disease (CHD) and musculoskeletal disorders
► Promote equal access to 'successful' services
► Meet national targets on healthcare priorities (eg CHD, mental health)

Will not do (2002/2003)
► Commission demonstrably ineffective services

US, major healthcare reform normally takes 10 years, because of what is generally recognized as its profound systemic impact on society as a whole. Few such cultural constraints yet apply in the UK where ruthless financial savings-driven general management in the modern NHS has often been justified by the speed of the organizational change it can deliver.

A depleted resource

This lack of relational awareness is self-evidently the case when moving the money around means either extra activity, as it did under the Conservative government from 1989 to 1997; or extra funds (and activity), as it does with the post-1997 Labour administration. In both cases the imperative is efficiency. More for less is the order of the day. The success of the Conservative government in, for the first time, directly linking NHS output levels to the changing level of financial inputs was demonstrated by the Treasury's automatic assumption of 2% annual NHS extra activity prior to any additional funds being allocated to the Department of Health in the public expenditure survey (PES) rounds of the early 1990s. Similarly, one of the current administration's earliest instructions to the NHS on 'changing the internal market' set unequivocal targets for efficiency through immediate reductions in bureaucracy by:

> 'reducing the cost of managing the NHS in 1997–98 by £100m, streamlining and reducing the flow of invoices to support this'
>
> (NHS Executive 1997a)

and deferring all new fundholding applications. The 'action plans' that followed in this letter from Alan Langlands, the NHS Chief Executive, set specific targets for cost reduction and in-year timetables. No mention is made of the contracting and clerical staff and practice managers, let alone the accountants affected. For many 'early retirement' or redeployment followed. For some the deliberately deferred central guidance on redundancy came too late in the summer of 1998 (NHS Executive 1998a). By the time the same year's *Priorities and Planning Guidance* was issued, just six executive letters later, the language in respect of risk management, service development and improved performance was entirely that of collaboration:

> *'Health authorities should work in partnership with NHS trusts and GPs to prepare . . . . the service and financial framework . . . The partners should adopt an open and transparent approach to sharing their financial position and prospects, to underpin constructive dialogue on the real issues and confirm agreement on the best way forward to meet local health needs'.*
>
> (NHS Executive 1997b)

These are fine words. Their context is that of the new three-year agreements signed up to by all local health agencies, with users, carers, clinicians and local authorities specifically listed for consultation. Efficiency is described as the 'sharing of support services', a very long way apparently from the separateness that was pervasive in the NHS internal market. There is just one real problem with all this. Working together on the financial resources would be so much more sustainable if the personal resources required for these new partnerships had been recognized. Throughout our work on the Relational Health Care (RHC) project we have had a sense of a policy as yet too 'good' (in terms both of ethics and capacity) for the NHS to deliver. Nowhere is this issue of deconditioning the 'old' NHS more apparent than in the confusion that now surrounds the role and contribution of competition in achieving improved efficiency through partnerships.

Competition

In terms of policy competition is taboo. You cannot find the word in health policy statements. Sometimes, as the 1999 Department of Health 10-year 'capital investment strategy' (Department of Health 1999a) nicely illustrates, this leads to some splendidly euphemistic phrasing. This strategy refers, for example, to:

> *'a single pot of unhypothecated resources . . . [which] will create greater flexibility for local authorities' investment decisions'.*

In a similar vein the stated central view is:

> *'that the Best Value regime will provide a framework for analysing the value for money of different public/independent sector mixes of service provision'.*
>
> (Department of Health 1999, pp44–5)

Competition continues despite the taboo

It is hard not to see this as being competition, at least on some occasions, in all but name; and as long as the separation of commissioning and providing responsibilities is sustained in the new NHS, then rivalry for the three-year service agreements is unavoidable. Competition is, therefore, at a minimum a latent factor in contemporary policy and its expression. For much of the NHS in 1999/2000, however, it remains much more than this. Behaviourally, competition is the basis on which most relationships have been created. It is the largest legacy of past experience for the encounters of the present day. It is the source of social and economic systems in large parts of 'middle England' where the pursuit of equality is regarded as an euphemistic sideshow. Particularly in primary care, competition has been the central *leit-motif* and this, in terms of patient recruitment and income generation, long pre-dates the advent of GP fundholding and the various primary care-led purchasing initiatives of the 1992–97 period. The contrast between the ideals of policy and the realities of practice in respect of competition has often been stark.

Competitive reality does not match collaborative ideals

The distance between central intentions and local implementation is actually still too wide. In conceptual and practical terms it currently constitutes a dishonest basis for the relationships of health. The case material presented at the RHC focus group on 'competition' during the 1998-engagement phase of the RHC project helped to illustrate this view. NHS regulations, for example, failed to offer protection to independent local pharmacists in the Manchester and Southampton areas who had developed a high-quality service, including domiciliary visiting, extended opening hours and practice-based prescribing protocols, when a multiple retailer, with its standard products and capacity to loss lead and lose overheads elsewhere in its operations, decided to make a commercially pre-emptive strike for premises in closer proximity to the GP surgeries.

The collaboration between two independent-sector nursing home providers in Hampshire came to an end when the combination of minimalist NHS inspection arrangements and a cost-cutting contracting culture in a local authority seeking to lower its own weekly contributions to continuing care, led to the larger organization opting out – leaving the local elderly residents with the one option and, in terms of cost and quality, the lowest option. In London we heard of competition between NHS hospitals for high fee-paying overseas patients. Income from these patients can be seen as helping us sustain both professional elites and their specialist research activities.

The result: winners and losers or excellence?

Competition for resources in the new NHS remains essentially competition with others. The relationship is a race:

- ▶ for the reputation of, for example, a 'beacon site'
- ▶ for influence not least over future resource allocation policies
- ▶ especially at PCG level, for financial resources themselves.

Competition is not yet, in behavioural terms, defined by the ends rather than the means. In each of the above examples the competition process is designed to produce winners and losers and the latter are not groups of NHS professionals and providers but their patients.

As the basis for relationships in the health system, this resource-based competition is clearly unacceptable and stems from the period in the NHS when the practice of competition was associated with such values as choice, autonomy and opportunity (eg NHS Executive 1996). What happens in the new NHS when a new family of values applies? Participation, cooperation, teamwork and quality are its members. Can competition belong here? Or is the new NHS really just substituting one form of competition for another – between such interorganizational units as health action zones and PCGs rather than between individual provider organizations, for example? Does competition apply as a motivating force only at the individual and group levels in healthcare; but not at that of the institution or system where interdependence is essential?

The policy stance of the Calman-Hines Cancer Services report can be pointed to in support of an affirmative response (Chief Medical Officers 1995). The rationale of specialist centres for exceptional cancer conditions supported by local units for the general mass of conditions was logical and seemingly irrefutable; so much so that some NHS Executive regional offices appeared to take an almost *laissez-faire* approach to this report's implementation. In practice they paid a price. Along the south coast, for example, every general hospital from Portsmouth to Plymouth at one point seemed to lay claim to a designated expert status. The private sector's use of competition:

> *'to encourage excellence by peer comparison where excellence is an end in itself and where pecuniary (or professional) reward is not the (sole) motivation . . . '*

> (Coleman D 1998, personal communication)

is an application of the concept which is still generally a stranger to NHS relationships.

Of course, there are exceptions. In East Wiltshire, we learnt of the expansion of a school nursing service previously threatened with extinction. It competed successfully on the basis of achieving local health prevention and promotion targets, which it helped to design. In Lambeth, Southwark and Lewisham we encountered a similar example where the service concerned was speech and language therapy and clients' social functioning the new currency of competition. In terms of resources the aims for competition are crucial. Their strength, clarity and conviction are all important. Without this integrity rules and regulations descend to the level simply of a game in which the pitch is for power and the competition is just for resources.

Integrity of purpose

To achieve this integrity of purpose in policy is tough in the new NHS. The recent scale of organizational turnover (p60) leaves a legacy not simply of relational damage but of personal and professional insecurity. This affects the allocation of resources themselves. The new government is less sure than it would like to be that, for example, the 'new deal' for nurses as part of 'securing a quality workforce' (NHS Executive 1998b) or the extra £2.1 billion for health arising from the 1998 central spending review (Department of Health 1999b) will produce their desired results.

This can become a self-fulfilling prophecy. For example, we have seen nursing schools, including that at Bournemouth University, which do not quickly achieve their increased student quotas face financial penalties which push them perversely towards alternative non-NHS contracts. Health authorities and NHS trusts with deficits in such affluent but, in terms of patients, demanding areas as Surrey and Berkshire, witness the additional funding only at distance through, for example, centrally-determined initiatives on healthy living centres, breast screening services and waiting lists. As a result the new resources make little discernible difference to baselines and even such innovations as NHS Direct – specifically designed to alleviate resource pressures – are regarded as both a distraction and potential source of new demand. The desired decentralization of resource management is experienced as the exact opposite and integrity of purpose is lost.

It is vital for the new NHS that it is both recovered and nurtured. Without it the relational potential of the health system cannot be released. This potential includes competition just as much as it does collaboration. The new NHS has tended to describe them as alternatives or even mutually exclusive in what was clearly an attempt to help create a new culture of new partnerships. Accordingly, at an early point in the Labour government's life the new Secretary of State for Health (1997) stated:

> 'There will be a 'third way' of running the NHS – a system based on partnership and driven by performance. It will go with the grain of recent efforts by NHS staff to overcome the obstacles of the internal market. Increasingly those working in primary care, NHS trusts and health authorities have tried to move away from outright competition towards a more collaborative approach. Inevitably, however, these efforts have been only partially successful and their benefits have not been as yet extended to patients in all parts of the country. This white paper (The New NHS: Modern, Dependable) will put that right. It will develop this more collaborative approach into a new system for the whole NHS.'

Competition and collaboration: the tactics of relationships

However, in the reality of relationships, competition is as inherent as collaboration. Both are automatic byproducts of the power produced by the imbalance of any social exchange (Blau 1967, Dawson 1996). We can after all collaborate to compete, as seen with the coming together of GP consortia to position themselves to achieve early NHS primary care trust (PCT) status (eg in North West Anglia). Also, we often compete to collaborate, as PCGs will testify from their experience of a multitude of recent approaches from pharmaceutical and life sciences companies regarding possible joint ventures.

For resources what matters is the relationships that apply either to collaborative or competitive approaches or a mixture of both. Competition can both divide and stimulate. Relationally, at least, it usually means increased contact. In the shire counties around London we have seen resource pressures further confirm the separation and underline the tension in the competitive relationships of individual general practices. In places like St Andrews and St Albans the converse has been true. Resource shortfalls have provoked the positive response of competing together for completely new sources of support, including European Union and urban regeneration funding, because of the prevailing strengths of inter-practice relationships. For collaboration the same applies:

in Swindon we heard it described as confirming the complacency of local provider relationships; in Wolverhampton, Leeds, Sheffield, Gosport and Fareham (and elsewhere), often under the auspices of local universities' outreach programmes, PCGs have ensured that local collaboration was at the heart of their inter-professional and cross-patch approaches to clinical governance.

In short collaboration and competition are the tactics of relationships. The real resource of relationships is their ends and the values they spawn for the ways in which competition, collaboration, and other tactical approaches are practised.

Table 3.2 is a practical illustration. The first version of this was prepared after a two-day RHC training programme for 25 facilitators of local PCG developments, held at Corpus Christi College in Cambridge during September 1998. Most of the participants were either trainers or management consultants. Most were self-employed, freelance or subcontractors for consultancy firms. They were less constrained than those in the NHS in addressing resource competition issues within the context of partnerships. Accordingly, the checklist they helped produce acknowledges that elements of competition are endemic at all levels in primary care and require recognition (eg via risk management and conflict resolution arrangements).

Moreover, for those working with the private sector, where the Cambridge attendees were accustomed to seeing competition even between major corporations confined to such areas as marketing and cost containment rather than the more fundamental areas of research and development and even production, these competitive elements could actually authentically be subsumed under the overall checklist heading of 'collaboration'. Such an approach allows the potential of intrinsically competitive functions to be released. For example, it can be argued that 'the new models of commissioning make the role of marketing more important' (Shelton and Miles 1999). The putting together of a health improvement programme (HImP) in this light has all the components of a classic marketing process, including the collation of competing needs and services, use of alternative feedback mechanisms and contestability on costs.

Table 3.3 was first designed and used by the PCGs in Northamptonshire. The three one-line statements of objectives distil the essential purpose of the new NHS for PCGs.

Table 3.2. Collaboration checklist for 2000/2001 time frame

Joint Unit	Objectives	Ways of working	Risk management	Conflict resolution
PCG/practice				
PCG/practices				
Intra-PCG				
PCG–PCG				
PCG–HA				

Please identify the key (problem) issues that the PCG must address to be viable.

Table 3.3. Role and resources of PCGs

Promote public health	£
Develop primary and community care	££
Commission secondary care	££££££
GP Fundholding in reverse!	

But the order, the £ signs and the 'punch line' convey an extremely powerful message for the integrity of purpose in the new NHS. Basic policy, aims and financial resources are not just out of alignment; they are the wrong way around. The purpose, accordingly, lacks integrity. Unless the relational resources for health and healthcare are more fully recognized, and used to shape NHS finances rather than the other way around, then this credibility gap will simply continue. It may even grow.

Rationing and rivalry

The RHC focus group on 'competition' described above worked on a dual analysis of the flash points for future competition and the potential benefits of rivalry in this competition, particularly at the level of PCGs, given the context and assumptions of sound relationships (Table 3.4). Interestingly in terms of resources, the rationing of treatments only came eighth in the assessment. The relational approach to competition seemed to suggest that this diminished as a specific issue the more it was located within an overall framework for addressing the imbalances of power in the contemporary NHS.

The benefits for resources utilization listed in Table 3.4 are impressive and they highlight the still important contribution of competition to the corporate goals of the new NHS – given the right relationships that can recognize and incorporate this. The 'last place' position of 'priorities for treatment' in Table 3.4 is, of course, completely at odds with the current conventional wisdom of NHS consultants and health-policy analysts (Honigsbaum *et al* 1995, Klein *et al* 1996). They predict rationing as the first future (if not present) issue requiring competitive and collective attention in the new NHS. In direct parallel with this line is that of central policy which, by contrast, places 'rationing' responsibilities directly with the individual relationships of GP and patient. Although the arrival of PCGs has helped share the burden a little, essentially this line has stayed the same between the last Conservative and the new Labour governments. The latter in looking to 'allow clinicians to influence the use of resources by aligning clinical and financial responsibilities' has actually instructed health authorities to move from Office of National Statistics (ONS) population data sources to GP registration lists in setting the baselines for PCG allocations (Department of Health 1998). The analysts accuse the politicians, whatever their affiliation, of ducking the issue. Their arguments are rooted in economics. In retaliation, ministers cloak themselves with the special 'personal' strength of UK primary care and little progress is made. For example, the split and sensationalized reaction to the essentially serious Sir Duncan Nichol-led enquiry into priority-setting alternatives served to sink it without trace within days if not hours of its publication (Nichol *et al* 1998).

Table 3.4. Competition: environmental analysis (source: RHC 'Competition' Focus Group, Sept 1998)

Resource 'hot spots'	can lead to	Resource utilization benefits
1 PCG versus PCG	→	1 New rewards and incentives to assess and address local health needs
2 NHS community trusts' survival	→	2 Value For Money skills substitution to enhance local special needs areas (eg low vision aids from optometrists, preschool screening by orthoptists)
3 Intra-PCG	→	3 More comprehensive skills mix at inter-practice levels
4 Control over HImPs	→	4 PCG commissioning to ensure convergence of health authority contracting and public health functions
5 Evidence-based (medicine) healthcare	→	5 Improved clinical process and outcome standards to regulate competition
6 Alternative philosophies of health and health care	→	6 Removal of barriers between public and non-public sector providers, opening up NHS to high status product development not just low status estate and facilities roles
7 Locality versus locality versus national agendas	→	7 Focus on quality to foster a culture of comparison and encouragement
8 Priorities for treatment	→	8 Wider participation and legitimacy of decision-taking processes

Against this background the relational perspective offers a more positive and productive way forward on the subject of prioritizing resources. The checklist analysis of the RHC focus group (Table 3.4) offers some pointers in terms of locating the issue within a wider framework. Revisiting the work of the Somerset Coast PCG, whose resource priorities are set out in Table 3.1, is also instructive as a characteristic illustration of the contribution PCGs can make. Using the relational profiling method (Table 7.1), this PCG undertook two assessments of the key relationships it would require to take forward its new resource management responsibilities over the next three years. An aggregated summary of its members' findings is set out in Table 3.5. It is broadly characteristic of how most PCGs see their position.

In many ways Table 3.5 represents as strong a relational profile as we have encountered in what is one of the most stable and competent parts of the NHS. The PCG members are confident in their purpose and roles and the Somerset Health Authority anticipates that all four PCGs in the county will reach NHS trust status by 2001. These are people worth listening to and learning from. For all their strengths they still scored at less than 50% in their relationships with social services and the public. District councils, the local media, education agencies and voluntary organizations did not even reach these scores. But, at the same time, it was these relationships that the PCG saw as crucial to legitimizing their future decision making. The explicit support of these agencies in 'rationing' will be crucial.

The PCG members near Weston-super-Mare recognized that the process of 'rationing' only really becomes viable if priorities are jointly owned, or better still are collective agreements, as well as being individual professional and personal decisions. They are better placed than anybody else in the health system to realize that too much

Table 3.5. Key PCG relationships beyond 1999/2000 (in order of significance)

Relationship subject	Relationship score (maximum of 25)
1 General practices/PCTs	19
2 Health authority	13
3 NHS trusts	13
4 Social services departments	12
5 The 'public'	8

can be loaded into the 'special' personal relationships of the GP and the patient. An holistic approach does not mean you can cover everything. A GP's three-times-a-year set of contacts of six to eight minutes each (or quite possibly less) has obvious limitations. The challenge is to translate the relationship strengths associated traditionally with primary medical care and convert them into those partnerships now required by primary care organizations which are acquiring wider responsibilities both for the commissioning of hospital services and the promotion of better community health.

If this analysis proves correct its implications are profound. It points directly to a much more 'localized' NHS, in which difficult decisions are embedded in a wider network of relationships with PCTs developing along the lines of the community organization and models (see p65–66). For this scenario to become a successful reality, the need for these relationships to be properly resourced is clearly paramount, which means having the right sort of strategies.

Summary

Relationships are much neglected by the NHS as a resource in both policy and practice. A more mature approach to relationships would legitimize as tactically appropriate a wider range of behaviours, including both collaboration and competition, to extend the potential resource base for healthcare. Primary care organizations are starting to recognize this, particularly as they look to gain local support on decisions regarding relative priorities. Integrity of purpose, however, remains an essential prerequisite in whatever way relationships are expressed.

References

Blau P (1967). *Exchange and Power in Social Life*. New York: John Wiley: 19–31.

Chief Medical Officers (1995). *The Future of Cancer Services*, Chief Medical Officers' report. London: Department of Health.

Dawson S (1996). *Analysing Organisations*. Basingstoke: Macmillan: 167–186.

Department of Health (1998). *The New NHS: Modern and Dependable. Guidance on Health Authority and Primary Care Groups*, HSC 1998/171 Wetherby: Department of Health: 3–10.

Department of Health (1999a). *Capital Investment Strategy for the Department of Health*. 15487, London: Department of Health.

Department of Health (1999b). *The Government's Expenditure Plans 1999–2000*. Cm 4203, London.

Honigsbaum F, Calltorp J, Ham C *et al* (1995). *Priority Setting Processes for Healthcare*. Oxford: Radcliffe Medical Press.

Klein R, Day P, Redmayne S (1996). *Managing Scarcity*. Buckingham: Open University Press.

NHS Executive (1996). *Primary Care: Choice and Opportunity*. London: Department of Health.

NHS Executive (1997a). *Changing the Internal Market*, EL (97) 33. Leeds: Department of Health: summary letter, para 3.

NHS Executive (1997b). *NHS Priorities and Planning Guidance 1998/99*, EL (97) 39. Leeds: Department of Health: annex, paras 5 and 6.

NHS Executive (1998a) *The New NHS: Modern and Dependable. Establishing Primary Care Groups*, HSC 1998/065. Leeds: NHS Executive: 16.

NHS Executive (1998b) *Working Together*, HSC 1998/162. NHS Executive, Leeds.

Nichol D *et al* (1998). *UK Health and Health Care Services – Challenges and Policy Options*. London: Health Care 2000.

Secretary of State for Health (1997). *The New NHS: Modern, Dependable*, Cm 3807 London; HMSO: 10–11.

Shelton P and Miles C (1999). External relations. *Health Management Journal* **Feb**: 22.

4
Strategy

'Though one may be overpowered,
two can defend themselves.
A cord of three strands is not quickly broken.'
(Ecclesiastes 4: 12)

Not just for planners

What is strategy?

Strategy can be a rather grandiose term for the decision making that comes with working in any organization. Decisions are ultimately about resource allocation. They will include issues surrounding service delivery: how and by whom are particular services best provided now and in the future? What are the priorities and should one service be cut in order to invest in another? They will affect the structure of the organization, its place in the local health economy, its staffing, its culture and the systems and processes that are developed. Strategy can have the positive connotations of foresight, direction, purpose and success. Strategy, in this sense, is important for all healthcare professionals because it represents their contribution to the effective long-term realization of the fundamental purposes of the NHS.

Strategy, however, also has many negative images. It can appear to be grandiose schemes for exceedingly modest outcomes: the unrealistic plans of remote bureaucracies, the flawed schemes of management consultants or resource-consuming consultation and mountains of paper which are out of date before they are (often not) implemented. Strategy, like much of the new NHS, is an ambiguous concept prompting ambivalent reactions. This uncertainty about strategy is captured in some of the comments expressed during the Relational Health Care (RHC) project:

'Strategy is something you do; and we don't implement!'

'The NHS thinks structure, structure, structure. It must think strategy, behaviour, structure.'

'Strategy is a waste of time. Policies and resources keep changing so there's not much point in long-term planning.'

'Strategy is vitally important so we can develop plans for the effects of long-term trends.'

'Strategy is about a direction of travel not a detailed map.'

'Strategy is about a blueprint for the district.'

The first quote [from a GP chair of a primary care group (PCG) board to a North Western Health Authority Executive Board] indicates one common problem with strategy: the lack of ownership and implementation. The second, from a Health Authority Chief Executive in South East England, indicates the concern that strategy too often lapses into structure. The last four of quotes came from a health authority in the South West NHS Region and vividly illustrate the very different views about strategy that may exist within an organization.

Uncertainty about strategy is not just a problem for the NHS. A review of the management literature over the past 40 years throws up very different definitions and theories and despite the wealth of literature it is still possible to find recent articles entitled 'What is strategy?' (eg Porter 1996). The main changes have been from internally-focused process engineering, to externally-focused planning designed to ensure competitive advantage, to soft systems approaches, to enhancing the capacity to be strategic. There are a number of important conclusions from this continuing debate about healthcare strategy.

Strategy is about success and organizational effectiveness

Strategy is defined with reference to the fundamental goals or purposes of an organization and the changes (or anticipated changes) in its environment which may affect its ability to achieve those goals. For businesses the goals are often seen in terms of competitive advantage and the means to this are increasingly described in relationship terms. So, for example, Waterman (1994) argues that:

> 'the key to competitive advantage is mainly this: building relationships with customers, suppliers and employees that are exceptionally hard for competitors to duplicate.'

For a public service such as the NHS, strategy will not be so closely linked to competitive advantage, but perhaps more towards effectiveness in achieving goals. These goals may be set externally (eg by policy) or internally. This means that there is no single health service strategy. There is a multilayered approach with different parts of the health service setting their own strategies. They will be interrelated (NHS organizations cannot ultimately ignore policy or each other), but they will not usually be fully coherent, especially as central policies do not always constitute a single unified strategy. So, for example, strategy for the primary care pilot may be about establishing its place in the local health system so that funding is continued after the pilot period. For the health authority it may be part of its public health strategy, while for the NHSE regional office it is part of the process of testing the delivery capacity of new organizational structures.

The nature of strategy is linked to the nature of the organization. In fact the links with other functions are broad as illustrated by the '7-S' model of organizational effectiveness (Waterman *et al* 1980). As Figure 4.1 illustrates, this sees strategy as just one of seven interconnected components of organizational effectiveness. Iles (1997, 48–53) has provided a helpful account of the use of this framework in the healthcare context. An illustration of the use of this framework in assessing the public health capacity of new forms of primary care organization is given on p51–54.

Strategy reflects the changing nature of health organizations and systems. Chapter 5 looks at the extent to which concepts of the virtual, stakeholder, community or learning organization are more appropriate for the new NHS than, for example, the traditional bureaucratic model of hierarchical structures and accountabilities. Organizational effectiveness in these contexts has much more to do with getting the relationships right and as a result creating effective decision making and delivery capacity, than laying the best five-year plans.

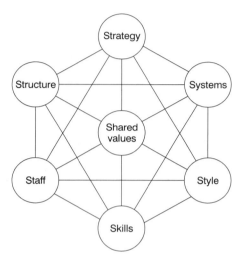

Strategy:	The actions that an organisation plans in response to, or anticipation of, changes in the external environment, customer needs and the strategies of competitiors.
Structure:	The means by which organisations divide up tasks and how they integrate and co-ordinate them.
Systems:	All of the porocedures, both formal and informal, that make the organisation 'work': budgeting, training, auditing, communicating, referral, assessment, discharge.
Staff:	The numbers and the kind of staff.
Skills:	The kind of skills required in health care organisations fall into four categories: clinical/technical; interpersonal; managerial; and research/reflection.
Style:	The way senior staff behave and what they value (in deeds, not just words).
Shared values:	The culture of the organisation, the beliefs that influence and motivate behaviour.

Figure 4.1. The 7-S framework [adapted from Iles (1997), pp51–53]

Strategy is inclusive, responsive and emergent

Strategy as rational planning, or a set of position statements which give rise to purchasing or capital investment plans, is now increasingly having to address the softer issues of strategic partnerships and processes. It is these soft issues which often prove hard to manage. Mintzberg (1988), in his account of the rise and fall of strategic planning, argues that planning should be seen as the operationalizing of strategy. This has been summarized by Clive Morton (an NHS trust chair) in terms of the three fallacies of strategic planning:

▶ its attempt at prediction in the era of discontinuity

▶ its typical detachment from operations

▶ formalized approaches do not forecast discontinuities (Morton 1998).

For an NHS in transition, which has experienced considerable organizational disconti-nuity; which seeks to put decision making as close to patients as possible and where future capacity will depend upon the very uncertain development of relationships, the limitations of planning become clear.

Responsiveness and inclusiveness go together: relationships cannot easily be controlled and attempting to do so is often counterproductive. The relational environ-ment is always changing and a strategy which depends upon relationships must there-fore be responsive to this environment. For the stakeholder organization, whose characteristics NHS organizations are increasingly expected to display through their openness and inclusiveness, a responsive strategy means more than simply looking at the external environment [by using PEST analyses (political, economic, social and tech-nological features of the external environment) or other tools] but 'engaging in system-atic dialogue with the networks of stakeholder relationships' (Wheeler and Sillanpää 1997, p132). Such an approach is important for reintegrating the NHS because:

> *'when we recognize that the environment is not separate from 'us', and that we do not necessarily have to compete or struggle against the environment, a completely new set of relationships becomes possible'.*

> (Wheeler D and Sillanpää

In working with many districts supporting PCG and health improvement programme (HImP) development the need for such new sets of relationships has been readily apparent. This relational approach also enables NHS organizations to shape their envi-ronment rather than be determined by it.

A consequence of this approach is that strategy is emergent, a term that corresponds well with our experiences of the strategic process for the NHS during the period of the RHC project. This is not a recipe for short termism. Indeed public health strategies, or major capital investment programmes, require a long-term view. Rather it is about creating organizations and strategic processes which can cope with change and contin-ually readjust strategies to achieve their long-term aims.

This emergent nature is reinforced by, for example, the focus on inclusive approaches to public health. As this expands the membership of the local health economy, strategy emerges from the latter's many interdependent relationships. This emergent characteristic, of course, does not make evidence-based planning redundant, but rather recognizes that this cannot be a fixed, unilateral process conducted in isola-tion from others. Strategy, and in particular a public health strategy, requires partici-pation in development and partnership in delivery. It must be responsive and inclusive – continually attuned to others' views and priorities and their capacities for successful delivery.

Inclusiveness in strategy then becomes important for a number of reasons. In the context of multisectoral, multi-agency approaches to delivering healthcare, the knowledge base and resources are diffuse. Accessing this knowledge, harnessing resources and ensuring the ownership and commitment that is needed to make significant progress require higher degrees of involvement. Inclusiveness is also a political issue: the legitimacy of strategy is increasingly seen in demonstrating both community and professional ownership.

Strategy should be efficient and effective

There are, of course, different degrees of ownership and involvement, and inclusiveness does not make leadership in strategy redundant. Our strategy simulations, particularly with groups of Masters degree students at the City University campus, have shown that the inclusive nature of Level 2 PCGs, for example, is not always matched by effective decision-making capacity. Strategy must be efficient and well directed, as well as inclusive. We have witnessed 'talking shops' that can waste resources without necessarily making better decisions or achieving greater commitment to delivery. In such cases those who are most vocal are not always the ones with most to contribute. In our experience of strategic processes some professionals have not always gained the hearing they deserve. In Camden and Islington, for example, in an illuminating exercise where 12 primary care professionals took it in turns to chair a 'mock' PCG meeting and invite contributions from each other with a view to improving local health, it was the local optometrist and community pharmacist who seemed to have the most to offer, but they were only chosen to speak at the ninth and tenth times of asking!

Strategy is about getting the relationships right – not just the structure

As always, the rhetoric of inclusive strategy is rather easier than the reality, not least because it requires changes in culture, behaviour and attitudes and not just formal processes. Policy can foster, or undermine, the conditions for effective strategy but it also depends on the individuals and organizations involved. The NHS can appear obsessed with structure. Indeed many of the people we have worked with fear that current policy will end up as another round of structural reform. As one health authority chief executive put it: 'the NHS thinks structure, structure, structure. It must think strategy, behaviour, structure'. Structures, however well designed both organizationally and in terms of fit with policy, may constrain the right behaviours or encourage the wrong behaviours. In a rapidly changing health environment they will not have the flexibility continually to adapt to external changes while preserving their internal relationships.

Developing a relational strategy

Strategy is, then, a fundamentally relational process. This is true for the financial aspects of strategy where risks and resources can be linked to relationships (see Chapter 3), as well as for more obviously relational dimensions such as public health partnerships. Strategy as planning, or as analysing and responding to the external environment, has well developed toolkits. The tools to support strategy as a relational process are much less well developed. In our work to support organizational and strategy development, the RHC project has used a framework for assessing relationships developed by the Relationships Foundation in Cambridge. The use of the tools for review purposes is described more fully in Chapter 8. Here we take one of our main projects (funded by the Health Education Authority) on how primary care organizations can improve public health as well as deliver healthcare as a more detailed case study of the relational aspects of strategy.

Public health provides a powerful example because HImPs are intended to be a core part of the strategic process. Many organizations, agencies and individuals have a stake in public health: the nature and quality of the relationships between them will be a significant factor in the development of effective and appropriate HImPs. The link between relationship and strategy can be seen as a cycle (Fig. 4.2). The process of strategy development is enabled by effective relationships but can also constitute a trigger for relationship development. The cycle may be virtuous or vicious: relationships, organizational development and public health strategy can be mutually reinforcing (which does not, of course, preclude encountering various crisis points), but can also become mutually destructive.

In developing a relational strategy there are two basic questions to consider: which relationships are involved (and important) and how strong or weak are those relationships? Relational development and review, which are also important parts of the overall strategic process, raise other questions which are addressed in Chapter 8. The simple exercise of mapping key relationships (see Fig. 7.1) is a useful first step. Identifying which relationships are essential for the strategic process, both now and in the future, and which are in particular need of development support, will help identify priorities for attention. There are hard choices here, both in terms of balancing the number of relationships that are maintained, and their depth, as well as disinvesting from some relationships in order to make time and resources available for other relationships which are becoming more important. For Porter (1996) the issue of

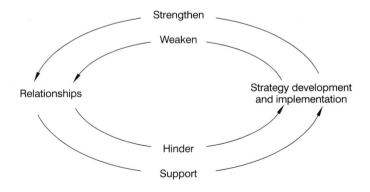

Figure 4.2. Relationships and strategy: a virtuous or vicious cycle

leadership in strategy is to make such choices – to establish the trade-off between activities that have no long-term competitive future (and, as Chapter 3 argues, competition remains important in the new NHS even if its focus has changed) and those that show promise.

The concept of a 'good' relationship can be misleading: apparently good relationships can, in fact, be complacent or collusive. Some conflictual relationships may be extremely robust, effectively dealing with the difficult and important issues. Nevertheless, gaining some indication of the strength of the relational basis to support health strategy is important in order to avoid initiating unsustainable processes which in the end run the risk of weakening the relationships further. Relationships are often perceived very differently by the parties to the relationship and these perception gaps are a good indicator of problems in the relationship.

Framework for assessing relationships

As we indicated earlier much of our work on supporting strategy has been based around a framework for assessing relationships developed by the Relationships Foundation (Schluter and Lee 1993, Scottish Prison Service 1995). There are many well established psychometric approaches for looking at interpersonal or team relationships, but diagnostics to support the development of relationships between organizations are much less well developed. Current approaches to social audit (Wheeler and Sillanpää 1997) provide some assessment of stakeholder relationships and assurance of management focus but are not principally designed to aid their development.

The approach adopted by the Relationships Foundation is to focus on the relational environment – which includes factors such as organizational structure and culture, work practices, infrastructure and skills – and the extent to which this creates the preconditions which will foster effective relationships. It is structured around five dimensions which are regarded as necessary, but not sufficient, conditions for effective relationships. As the approach does not presuppose a particular model of a 'good' relationship, the weighting attached to each dimension, and its particular focus, varies according to the kind of relationship and the particular context. The nature of the relationships between a patient and a practice nurse or an NHS Direct nurse, or with a GP as opposed to an Accident and Emergency unit's consultant, may be quite different. Different aspects of the relationship, or different outcomes, may be seen as more important and therefore greater importance may be attached to different preconditions in order to ensure that these outcomes are achieved.

This approach was initially developed in the context of work for the Scottish Prison Service. As well as our work in the health service it has also been further developed by the Relationships Foundation in partnership with KPMG, the management consultants, for use in the business context. The focus until now has been on supporting relationship development. It does not, as yet, provide a fully validated measure of relationships. Indeed, as we argue in Chapter 8, there are many methodological obstacles to doing so. In the course of widespread use it has, however, proved effective and helpful in crystallizing key issues and in enabling constructive discussion. The elements of the framework have been developed and refined through research as well as the experience of working with many organizations in a wide range of contexts.

There are of course many possible ways of classifying and analysing relationships. The one set out in Table 4.1 has proved useful for us, accessible for participants and able to accommodate the wide range of potential factors that may affect interorganizational relationships.

Commonality – valuing similarity and difference

Commonality enables individuals and organizations to work together towards shared goals. While tensions can be creative, and there may be differences in roles and responsibilities, if these are not set in the context of some shared objectives and understanding, then the likelihood of performance-hindering conflict may be increased. Common objectives provide the basis for working together. Without real, shared and defined objectives (as opposed to generalized goals) organizations or teams may end up pulling in different directions or come into conflict over priorities. Agreement over the means of achieving goals may be as important as agreement about the goals themselves. The process by which agreement on objectives is reached is important in building commonality. Many of the strategic processes we have witnessed have been hampered by differing views of health (and local health priorities) as well as competing organizational interests.

Shared culture reduces the risk of misunderstandings, difficulty in articulating shared objectives and the lack of a shared basis for resolving differences of opinion. This applies both to professional and organizational cultures. A sense of common identity, of ultimately being in the same boat, can reflect the strength of the relationship as well as providing a basis for its development. This may be expressed through establishing some common culture or through developing working practices which take account of different cultures rather than just working round them or simply ignoring them. Commonality does not require uniformity. Differences can add value to a relationship although it is important that they are seen as enriching the relationship and not just as obstacles to be overcome. The way in which disagreements are handled is also important: their resolution can strengthen commonality or may only seek to reinforce the differences. Different professional and organizational cultures in the contemporary NHS have been a frequent problem, engendering misunderstanding, mistrust and competing interests.

Parity – use and abuse of power

Parity does not mean equality in a relationship. Authority, influence or rewards in a relationship may rightly vary, although it is important that differentials are accepted and not abused. It is rarely a simple picture, for there are many different kinds of power

Table 4.1. Framework for assessing relationships

▶	Commonality	– valuing similarity and difference
▶	Parity	– use and abuse of power
▶	Multiplexity	– breadth of knowledge
▶	Continuity	– shared time over time
▶	Directness	– quality of the communication process

(financial control, regulatory or sapiential authority, political influence, control of delivery, or exit and veto rights) in a relationship, and different parties in a relationship are likely to have different kinds of power.

Parity requires, and is fostered by, participation and involvement which ensure that people have some real say in decisions that affect their work. Lack of participation may mean that strategic objectives are not owned, reduce morale and stifle innovation. Inadequate influence in a relationship with respect to tasks or responsibilities is a frequent source of frustration.

The fairness of benefits in a relationship can engender cooperation and foster commitment to a relationship from which both parties can benefit. 'Win–win' relationships where the benefits are identified and clearly communicated are more likely to be successful, even if the gains for the two sides are not the same. The presumption of altruism is an inadequate basis for collaboration (Hudson 1998). Fair conduct in the relationship is necessary for trust and respect. The lack of this was frequently cited as a major obstacle to effective collaboration by those project participants whose experience of inter-professional relationships has not always been characterized by mutual respect. Double standards, prejudice and favouritism are extremely corrosive.

Perceptions of parity often vary considerably – it is hard to find anyone in the NHS who feels they hold power in their key strategic relationships. It is common to find both parties vulnerable and disempowered although this mutuality is not always recognized. Trust, confidence and commitment are the casualties.

Multiplexity – breadth of knowledge

Multiplexity looks at the breadth of the relationship. This can enhance mutual understanding and enable a broader appreciation of the range of skills and experience that individuals or organizations can contribute. It helps avoid strategies which ignore the realities of the underlying relationships and may open up new opportunities that arise from unsuspected common ground or unrecognized resources. Knowledge of a counterpart's organization or department is important to appreciate the constraints under which they work, to identify shared objectives and to develop appropriate ways of joint working. Knowledge of role or skills is important for the effectiveness of joint work and helps avoid flawed assumptions or misunderstandings, missed opportunities or suboptimal resource utilization. Knowledge of the person (such as his or her interests or values) can strengthen the relationship and aid its management.

For project participants multiplexity has consistently been an uncertain dimension of the relationship. It has perhaps been most evident in the mutual ignorance of NHS and local authority staff about each others' organizations. Failure to understand different decision-making processes, structures, and ways of working are seen as major problems in partnership working around HImPs. For the new strategic relationships there is much groundwork still to be done.

Continuity – shared time over time

Time is the currency of relationships. The continuity of contact over a period of time provides the opportunity for both individual and organizational relationships to develop, although difficult decisions may need to be made about which relationships to invest time in. When time is actually invested in a relationship is also important: time invested at the start of a relationship can avoid time-consuming problems downstream.

The length and stability of the relationship over time creates the opportunity for individual rapport and improved mutual understanding to develop, as well as providing a context for long-term issues to be addressed at an organizational level. Where staff turnover is high – as we have found in many parts of the local NHS in London – locking in the benefits of individual and informal relationships to create an organizational history and overview of the relationship is often important. Managing change in the relationship is important if such benefits of change as career progression and bringing in new people are to be achieved without undermining the quality and effectiveness of existing relationships.

A lack of continuity has been a pervasive experience throughout this project. Although time has been pressured for most people, their principal concern has not been the amount of contact. Rather it has been the legacy of change and the impact of staff turnover. Doctors have often been seen as a focus for continuity within local healthcare systems. A number of participating doctors, however, were concerned that their junior colleagues would be more mobile, diminishing this resource. There was also some frustration, particularly in NHS trusts, with staff turnover in health authorities: precious time was invested in 'training' staff to understand services and they then moved on. Too much discontinuity may erode the willingness to commit to and invest in relationships, to the detriment of future strategic processes.

Directness – quality of the communication process

Directness influences the quality of communication in the relationship. The medium of communication affects the amount and quality of information exchanged. Face-to-face communication, for example, allows non-verbal signals to be picked up and immediate responses to be made, so enabling better understanding. It is perhaps of particular importance for difficult or particularly important issues. It is, however, resource intensive so it is important to ensure that the right medium is used at the right time. The channel of communication influences both the quality and efficiency of information exchange. Both can be reduced if channels are blocked or if information and decisions are too often received second-hand, via messages or through several levels of bureaucracy. Accessibility and responsiveness are key issues here.

Communication style and skills are also significant. The structure of the communication must be complemented by the right behaviour. For instance, a lack of openness can impede trust and undermine partnership. A cycle operates: openness can create trust and trust can encourage openness, but a downward spiral of decreased trust and impaired communication can also develop.

Relational strategy: the baseline

Making strategy a relational process will represent a big change in terms of who is involved, the focus of strategy (increasingly driven by the pursuit of public health) and the nature of the process. An indication of the magnitude of this change comes from our 1997–99 project for the Health Education Authority (HEA) looking at how primary care organizations can improve public health as well as deliver healthcare. The following account is based on a report for the HEA (Meads *et al* 1999) and is reproduced with its permission.

Public health strategies

Looking at the starting points we do not have to go back very far to find strategies which were principally about practice development or secondary care purchasing. Public health was not a major feature of strategy. This is acknowledged in central policy statements:

> 'The HoN [Health of the Nation] was seen by those in primary care as 'someone else's agenda', and as irrelevant because of its population focus, long time-scales and emphasis on non-medical interventions – all features which were opposite in character to the traditional GP practice'.
>
> (Department of Health 1998)

The HEA project started six months before the publication of the green paper *Our Healthier Nation* (Secretary of State for Health 1998). An initial stocktake of health strategies revealed very different starting points with great variation between health authorities and between primary care organizations in their approaches to strategy; understanding of the health improvement agenda; processes by which they agreed priorities and experience of the process.

This is not surprising as PCGs, which were then in the process of formation, are not *de novo* creations. Their diverse nature and development experience are significantly influenced by the legacy of the differing ways and speeds in which previous national policies have been implemented, as well as by the wide range of specific local factors and contexts. These include the nature of the local community, its health status, boundaries and political structures, relationships with other NHS and non-NHS organizations, and the particular individuals involved. PCGs' capacity to improve public health as well as deliver effective healthcare in the future will depend on the extent to which these legacies can either be built on or overcome. Arguably, authentic primary healthcare has to be much more a local cultural development than a central policy product.

Initially strategies were seen in very different terms, with some health authorities in fact describing service development strategies or aggregated local provider plans rather than broader approaches to improving health through multi-agency working. Some primary care organizations, on the other hand, described their practice development or business plans. The extent to which strategies were known about also varied. In an earlier RHC project looking at the relationship between a health authority and a NHS community trust in central London, many trust staff perceived the health authority as more short termist than them. On discussion it emerged that there was a five-year strategy, but it had not been circulated to many trust staff, let alone read by them, and decisions which affected them were not clearly linked back to the longer-term strategy.

Priorities in the health strategies also varied widely, with approaches to priority setting often reflecting local organizational history rather more than local health needs. Health authorities talked about having taken a broad partnership approach to priority setting but on closer investigation this was often limited to brief consultation with local social service departments or multidisciplinary approaches informed mostly by health professionals. Primary care organizations admitted to 'GP anecdote and day-to-day experience' as well as feedback from providers about pressures. Some health authorities were primarily reactive with priorities set in response to national pressures, local pressures from service providers and users, or social services budgetary constraints. Others were more proactive with local stakeholder workshops and forums.

The supporting relationships

The second part of the baseline assessment was to examine whether the relationships were in place to support both the development and delivery of health strategies. The challenge for PCGs lies in the fact the development and delivery of a public health strategy depends upon a wide range of relationships which may be new relationships, different kinds of relationship, or previously neglected or difficult relationships. In some areas health strategies are being built on a strong relational base. So, for example, some primary care organizations had established relationships with local authorities (eg via neighbourhood nursing teams coterminous with local authority community action forums), while for others these are substantially new relationships to be created.

The assessment focused initially on the relationship between participants in the health authorities and primary care organizations with lead responsibility for public health. We found wide variation in the relationships reflecting differing stages of development in response to earlier policies, local geography and politics, previous experience of joint working and the impact of other external relationships. Despite the diversity of starting points and satisfaction with relationships, a number of common issues emerged (Table 4.2). Behind these key issues lay significant differences in expectations and perceptions of the relationship.

Commonality was in many cases the weakest aspect of the relationship. A lack of commonality was presumed in some cases, eg a belief by health authority staff that GPs were not interested in public health. Such stereotyped views meant that significant areas of common ground had gone unrecognized. While different health ideologies were thought to be a problem in the relationship, this was not a major issue between individual participants. There were, however, widespread doubts among participating GPs about how easy it would be to bring colleagues fully on board with them.

There were significant differences in professional cultures, health ideologies and organizational priorities. In many cases these were seen as obstacles to progress with considerable scepticism about whether they could easily be overcome. Those involved in the relationships had built up a degree of shared understanding and objectives, although this was sometimes more around operational than strategic issues. Real shared objectives were only gradually emerging: in many cases this was a consequence of the inadequacies of earlier consultation processes which had failed to secure adequate ownership of the strategies and priorities that emerged. Links between local priorities and health authority-wide priorities were also insufficient.

Table 4.2. Common themes in health authority/primary care organization relationships

- ▶ Superficially good relationships could conceal failure to address important but difficult strategic issues
- ▶ Rational planning had produced good strategies but without the processes to secure buy in – adequacy of consultation was perceived very differently
- ▶ Increased participation by general practices was best gained by promoting the practical advantages, not just the future vision
- ▶ Health authority automatic assumption of local leadership roles and consequent conduct of the relationship caused resentment. Inclusive leadership was felt to be key to future progress
- ▶ Conflicting organizational priorities and interests hindered the relationship in all cases
- ▶ There was also greater common interest than most participants initially recognized
- ▶ Professional defensiveness and lack of mutual understanding inhibited progress in a number of cases.

During the course of the project uncertainty about the changing role of health authorities (eg as facilitator, power-broker or regulator) and their future prospects caused uncertainty about the extent to which common purpose was attainable. In the London NHS Region some have taken the NHS Executive's announcement that it does not anticipate any health authority mergers for three years to mean that all health authorities have less than four years to go. The extent to which health authorities were, or were perceived to be, creating distance in the relationship to strengthen accountability and protect all stakeholder interests, defending their own organizational interests, or working closely together with new primary care organizations to ensure the effective implementation of new policies, influenced the nature and extent of the common ground that was expected.

There were some unifying forces. In some cases it was a 'common enemy' such as an overspending acute trust. Where a major part of the public health role was managing this demand, there were wide variations in the extent to which those in primary care recognized this as being to their benefit rather than perceiving the lower involvement in primary care as a lack of interest. While this was tactically effective in bringing organizations together, it is unlikely to prove an adequate foundation for developing and implementing public health strategies in the long term, particularly where the 'enemy' is an important part of the strategy equation. The attempts of primary care organizations in Southampton, for example, to see overspends as a shared problem to be resolved to mutual benefit may be more productive in the long term. Establishing a strong sense of shared accountability, either to the local community or failing that to the centre, is also likely to be important. A broader focus such as city-wide initiatives could also help bring people together as we witnessed in Leeds, Sheffield and Nottingham where unitary local authorities play significant parts in reinforcing this perspective. Future central policies should perhaps also have an important role to play in giving incentive to the development of commonality.

In terms of building this aspect of the foundations for a relationship a number of direct imperatives emerged:

- ▶ identify the common ground that does exist to enable early wins (this included integrating other practices)

- ▶ recognize that there are no short cuts to cultural change – start by working with the other's culture rather than threatening it

▶ the need for inclusive leadership to establish commonality

▶ building commonality at a personal level could enable organizational obstacles to be overcome more easily.

Issues of power in the relationship were complex, with it again being common for all parties to feel disempowered. This reflected the different kinds of power operating in the relationship as well as the influence of other relationships. Thus, one health authority felt disempowered by the uncertainty surrounding what future central guidance might contain and the uncertainty about its future role, while its primary care organizations were frustrated by the health authority's continuing presumption of the local leadership role and the right to make (in the view of the primary care organization) unilateral decisions. Divergent expectations and perceptions about leadership and decision making were a major source of friction in the relationship. Responsibility and accountability were out of alignment, with nationally-imposed tight timetables and, in some cases, local divisions constraining effective consultation. Differing expectations of future change led to differing views of how roles should develop. Issues of parity between health professionals were not a focus of this project but were an influential background factor, particularly during the election of PCG board members.

There was considerable uncertainty as to the extent to which there was good mutual understanding of each other's organizations, their individual skills and interests and the particular pressures and constraints with which each had to work. Myths and stereotypes affecting attitudes and belief in the potential of the relationships meant that significant areas of common ground were, in some cases, unrecognized. Opportunities for progress had been missed as a result. The limited breadth in the relationship was partly a consequence of the communication pattern. Where much of the contact had been around operational issues or formal consultation processes there had been few opportunities to build a broader understanding of each other's work or organizations. Having public health professionals with a background in general practice was seen to be helpful in enabling this understanding to be built up. For example, in both North-West Anglia and West Hertfordshire, where considerable progress has been made in the strategic processes for public health improvement, the Directors of Public Health each have substantial experience as GPs.

Continuity was regarded more as a pervasive background problem, rather than a specific feature of the relationships between health authorities and primary care organizations. Individuals had in most cases known each other for several years and had developed good personal working relationships. A period of constant organizational change meant that these had not necessarily translated into good organizational relationships. For one participating organization the average lifetime of a job was 18 months, with there being, on average, two postholders during this period. Investment in relationships was perceived to be time well spent, although not always easy to achieve.

There was universal agreement that not enough attention was devoted to long-term issues affecting the relationship. This was partly a consequence of the immediate pressures of policy implementation deadlines. Both health authorities and primary care organizations hoped that once the immediate pressure of PCG implementation had passed there would be more opportunities to address long-term issues, although there was also a recognition that there were always pressures which hampered long-term thinking.

Communication channels appeared to be reasonably effective. In some cases there were concerns about the prevalence of hidden agendas and uncertainty about what counterparts really thought. In most cases the participants represented the most developed aspects of health authorities' relationships with primary care organizations. It is likely that these were not necessarily typical of the majority of local relationships, where levels of contact, trust and directness may well be lower.

Indeed the HEA project participants were thought to represent the top end of the relational spectrum. They were from leading-edge sites, with a history of working together and often well-developed personal relationships. Yet even with a reasonably strong relational base the pressures of PCG implementation caused some tensions. The prospects for health strategy where the relationships were less well developed were thought to be far less promising.

Relational strategy – future prospects

In our work with PCGs we have identified four organizational types (Table 4.3):

▶ *Defence association:* characterized by resistance to change and the staunch advocacy of the relationship between the professional and individual patients.

▶ *Friendly society:* matches most closely to the Level 2 PCGs. They are inclusive and, initially, enjoyable, but ultimately frustrating as talk outstrips action; They are also inefficient as the nature of the inclusive processes is costly in terms both of time and money.

▶ *Executive agency:* efficient and effective, but without a public health focus. Contracting and negotiating skills are harnessed to deliver specific services, but the change agenda is internally defined.

▶ *Franchised company.* There are currently few organizational developments with a comprehensive approach to assuming a franchised responsibility for the local population's health and healthcare, but this was the aspiration for many of the districts where we have worked.

Each of these organizational models has different capacities for developing effective health strategy and will approach it in different ways. These differences are clearly illustrated in the outcomes from a simulation with project participants to apply an analytical framework designed to identify the seven dimensions of a well integrated organization (see Fig. 4.1). The outcomes of the strategy component are set out below [extracts from Meads *et al* (1999) are reproduced below with permission].

Defence association

For the defence association public health strategy is external to PCGs and driven by the health authority. Priorities are more likely to be meaningful at practice than PCG board

Table 4.3. Characteristics of four organizational PCG types [Source: Meads et al (1999), p36]

Type	A Defence association	B Friendly society	C Executive agency	D Franchised company
Status	Professional network	HA subcommittee	Brokers/firm	Mixed status public utility
Accountability (to)	DoH/GPC	HA/LMC	Trusts	National/regional regulators
Purpose	To advocate and represent individual general practices' interests for growth and survival	To encourage an inclusive approach to local health issues, based on existing practice arrangements	To contrain secondary care and redirect resources to practices	To control majority of healthcare resources of local population and seek a health dividend
Objectives	To sustain GMS income	To support HA as principal purchaser of healthcare	To release critical mass of GPs for general medical practice	To operate as a corporate organization in terms of investment and savings
	To preserve practice configuration	To promote primary care teams with GP leadership	To set direction for community health services	To address population and individual health issues in balance
	To defend professional autonomy	To explore opportunities for inter-practice collaboration	To improve scope for improved skills substitution and inter-professional working	To gain community acceptance and active endorsement
	To respond effectively to local consultations on health issues	To maintain district as NHS performance unit	To resolve secondary/primary care conflicts via interclinician deals and trade-offs	Radically to revise both GMS and HCHS working practices
Management (by)	Liaison GPs and HA middle manager links	Commissioning (non-GPFH) GPs plus HA purchasing/corporate services managers	Former GPFH leads and managers – from practices and trusts	Senior community trust or HA executives, plus 'new' primary care professional leads on primary health care
Health strategy	Operational responses to nationally determined policies and contracts	Derived from DPH annual report and profiles of patient demand, augmented by effective individual representations	Intermediate care based – avoidable A&Es, continuing care, acute episodes, etc. Influenced by SSD community care plans	Based on patient enrolment principle – registered population signed up to organization's health and business priorities – as described in trust prospectus
Public health (function)	Very limited personnel resources, focused on core roles of communicable diseases, HNAs, etc	Operationally aligned with HA commissioning directorate. Closely involved in secondary care and clinical effectiveness issues	Promoting public health issues and alliances at strategic levels with unitary authorities or commerce, etc via shared SLAs	Split between overall performance monitoring and outposted advisory roles; leading multiprofessional public health networks including health visitors
Information	Extrapolated from national data sources (eg ONS DoH, MDs)	Locality analyses at parish/ward levels by HA based on NHS morbidity and hospital referral categories	Combined with LAs and based on district council/municipal boundaries; including CHS profiles	Built up from practice-level health needs assessments and combined with information sources of three other PCO types, plus literature/research findings
Internal relations (key)	Individual GP-based, with small and single-handed practices prominent. Strong support from practice administrative staff	Inter-practice forums and committees (eg audit, PGE), plus HA functions for contracting/commissioning	Paramedical staff; full range of community nursing, 'lead' GPs	Subject of minimal attention – real risks of implosion
External relations (key)	GPC; individual patients, traditional NHS managers, RCGP (national)	HA members and chief executive, prescribing adviser, primary care alliance, RCGP (regions); hospital consultants	Community trust service clinicians and managers, social services, budget managers, health economists, accountants, voluntary organizations, Association for Primary Care	New PCTs national group, NICE/CH1, regional offices/assemblies, media and politicians, commercial sector, major providers
Organizational prospects	Limited life expectancy	Transitional	Temporary	Fragile basis for future organizational development

CHI = Commission for Health Improvement, CHS = community health services, DoH = Department of Health, DPH = director of public health, GMS = general medical services, GPC = general practice committee, GPFH = general practice fundholder, HA = health authority, HCHS = hospital and community health services, HNA = health needs assessment, LA = local authority, LMC = local medical committee, MDS = minimum data set, NICE = National Institute for Clinical Excellence, ONS = Office of National Statistics, PCO = primary care organization, PCT = primary care trust, PGE = postgraduate education, RCGP = Royal College of General Practitioners, SLA = service level agreement, SSD = social services directorate

level and reflect nationally set priorities, financial incentives and main areas of dissatisfaction with current service provision. However, from the health authority perspective, health strategy may be focused more on promoting the organizational development and hence long-term strategic capacity of the PCG, although it may not want a full NHS trust to develop so that it can retain control. In some cases there may be potential to bypass the PCG and focus on alternative change agents such as health action zones. Overall a lack of senior level health authority involvement in PCGs suggests that they are not the key to the health authority's public health strategy.

While recognizing that the majority of medical practitioners in this type of organization subscribe to a medical model of health, there is a danger in underestimating their interest in public health. Working with, or appearing to impose, a very different social model of health is likely to appear threatening and counterproductive. Initially it seems best to work with the medical model and to demonstrate the medical benefits to patients of an improved public health strategy.

Changing attitudes, culture and health ideologies need to be part of any strategy for developing greater public health involvement. There are no short cuts to this process – significant progress can be expected to take around two years. Composition of the PCG is a key catalyst for change: lay members and other health professionals can provide the opportunity to filter in different perspectives and initiate partnerships. Where local networks develop they need effective health authority support to ensure they become a platform for future progress. Clinical governance with its associated peer pressure can be an important entry point to encourage more corporate thinking and strategic capacity. It can also, of course, be a major threat to conventional wisdom and professional pride.

Friendly society

The friendly society is very inclusive in its approach (that is including the views of all individual members – the whole primary care team). It wants to move forward from this organizational position but is unclear how it will do this or what it wishes to achieve. Some of the GPs in this model have been working as a 'locality' group, 'co-commissioning' (in theory) with the health authority – although in reality the latter has made the major commissioning decisions in the past. The health authority's views are accepted as an accurate reflection of local health needs although it is not clear whether or not they are 'evidence-based' and the PCG may want to challenge these as it becomes more established. The friendly society, therefore, begins by thinking about access to services, rather than wider inequalities in health status. In terms of multi-agency work, there is no local strategic focus for this; joint health strategies have been very much at a high organizational level – between the health authorities and local authorities.

Executive agency

The executive agency's strategy is pragmatic, selective and focused. The approach is based on 'doing deals' between clinicians with the positional power and personal influence both to change clinical practice and carry professional colleagues with them. Accordingly, the strategy of addressing head on major rather than marginal targets for secondary to primary care transfers (eg A&E rather than maternity) is underpinned by a readiness to constrain GP referrals so that these resource shifts are not jeopardized. This is a health service rather than a health strategy.

Franchised company

The franchised company has the most comprehensive health strategy of the four organizational types. Its mission is to improve the health and wellbeing of the population and to reduce health inequalities and social exclusion. This language is important at this level because it incorporates the roles (and expectations) of both the Department of Health and local government, focusing on 'inequalities' as a joint and shared priority. It means the organization's need to engage in a bottom-up approach to assessing needs and selecting priorities and therefore to questioning 'old priorities'. The actual process of engaging communities is paramount. It is based on a range of methods which recognize the natural communities which make up the population and can include whole systems approaches, focus groups and citizens juries.

Its specific strategies for priority areas span the full continuum of needs of population groups to improve their health and wellbeing, ie health services, local government services and community development. For example, plans for older people cover hip replacements, community safety, transport, housing, heating and social networks.

Its planning is based on the totality of NHS and local government resources and expenditure for the PCG population, plus an awareness of the possible resources available in other sectors. It uses sophisticated programme planning techniques, eg health impact assessment analysis, to enable alternative investment strategies to be tested. All stakeholders, including communities, participate in debates about investment and rationing decisions. There is an increased awareness and ownership of resource consequences of investment choices. Balanced judgements that recognize the need to meet certain national standards and requirements as well as respond to local priorities characterize this level, as do different styles of service provision. The design and delivery of services based on new ways of involving families, individuals and communities include delegated budgets to communities, advocacy for isolated/vulnerable groups and support for an infrastructure of community groups.

Concerned with ensuring that wider policies and strategies operate to promote the health and wellbeing of the local communities and address inequalities, this organization tests the boundaries of regulations and seeks freedoms to operate in more integrated and flexible ways. It recognizes the need to ensure that quality standards and effective practice are adopted, eg via the National Institute for Clinical Excellence (NICE), and that standards are universally available to socially-excluded groups.

Change of culture

Each of the following represents a challenging vision for the future of the NHS:

- ▶ focusing on strategy and not just structure
- ▶ putting public health at the heart of health strategy
- ▶ getting the relationships right successfully to develop and implement strategies.

Success is far from guaranteed for any of them, as our research findings outlined above in the HEA programme on new primary care organizations and public health illustrate.

In much of the NHS there is a passionate desire to do better for patients and real frustration with inadequacies of some current service provision or inefficiencies in the system. (There is also, in places, unjustified complacency.) Yet alongside this there is widespread tiredness and uncertainty. Strategy should be something to get excited about. It should give people a voice and encourage real participation. It should ensure that provision is aligned with needs and prompt the development of structures, systems, processes and behaviours to enable more effective delivery of healthcare. Yet much of the energy for health strategy currently lies outside the NHS: participants from local authorities and management consultancies, for example, contributing with more self-confidence and, at times, greater vision.

Without proposed cultural change strategy will lapse into structure and dynamism into fossilization. Strategy requires living with change and continually readjusting to the wider health economy rather than creating structures to keep change at bay. The old securities (if they ever in fact existed) of control and stability must be, in part, exchanged for the security that comes from robust partnerships, community legitimacy and acknowledged success and quality in delivery. Strategy in the new NHS is thus far more than simply a different process for decision making and planning. It represents a fundamental change of culture.

Such change is never easily made. It is made more difficult where the underlying relationships are weak and where there is so much uncertainty about roles, influence and agendas. For health strategy the greatest opportunities often coincide with the greatest perceived threats. Many of these are linked with new organizational developments. But it is only by rising to these opportunities that long-standing concerns about healthcare delivery can be addressed.

Summary

Strategy should be an inclusive, responsive and effective process for making the choices that are part and parcel of any organization's efforts to fulfil its fundamental purposes. It is not just for planners, but 'belongs where the action is'. Developing and implementing strategies depends upon relationships, but the new NHS runs the risk of pursuing strategies which outstrip their relationship basis. Public health strategies provide a clear and powerful illustration of this. Strategy in the new NHS is more than simply a different process for decision making and planning. Emergent strategies and fluid organizational developments require a significant cultural change as well as new forms of security and confidence that come from robust partnerships, community legitimacy and acknowledged success and quality in delivery. Without it strategy will lapse into structure.

References

Department of Health (1998). *The Health of the Nation: A Policy Assessed*. London: HMSO.
Hudson R (1998). *Primary Care and Social Care*. Leeds: Nuffield Institute.
Iles V (1997). *Really Managing Health Care*. Buckingham: Open University Press.

Meads G, Killoran A, Ashcroft J, Cornish Y (1999). *Mixing Oil and Water*. London: Health Education Authority.

Mintzberg H (1988). *The Rise and Fall of Strategic Planning*. Hemel Hempstead: Prentice-Hall.

Morton C (1998). *Beyond World Class*. Basingstoke: Macmillan Business: 187.

Porter M (1996). What is strategy? *Harvard Business Review* **Nov/Dec**.

Schluter M and Lee D (1993). *The R Factor*. London: Hodder and Stoughton.

Scottish Prison Service (1995). *Relational Prison Audits*, Occasional Paper No. 2. Edinburgh

Secretary of State for Health (1988). *Our Healthier Nation*. London: HMSO.

Waterman R (1994). *The Frontiers of Excellence: Learning from Companies that Put People First*. London: Nicholas Brealey Publishing: 170.

Waterman R, Peters T, Phillips J (1980). The 7-S framework. In: Quinn JB and Mintzberg H, eds. *The Strategy Process*. Englewood Cliffs, New Jersey: Prentice-Hall, 309–14.

Wheeler D and Sillanpää M (1997). *The Stakeholder Corporation*. London: Pitman Publishing.

5
Organization

'Is there anything of which one can say,
'Look! This is something new?'
It was here already, long ago;
it was here before our time.'
(Ecclesiastes 1: 10)

Theory and practice

The pace of change in organizational practice has now left much of organizational theory behind. This is a problem, particularly for those with responsibilities for implementing central policy. Organizations have long been the preferred vehicle for the delivery of policy and organizational restructuring the favourite option for adjusting that delivery. The problem now is that this approach is no longer reliable. Organizations are not what they were; the changes required are more than just adjustments; and the theory no longer applies.

Hierarchy in theory

Any literature survey of organizational theory and research will still be characterized by some simple biases. Most of it is based in the US. Not much of substance, and certainly very little with detachment, has been written since 1990, and much of the theory remains based on either international corporations or production-based private companies. For the public sector, worthy but now hopelessly simplistic organizational theories are still taught. On the one hand there is the classic bureaucratic model of hierarchic accountabilities and spans of control (Weber 1947), which could be applied to the NHS when it was a set of closed institutions but not to the modern military let alone the complex networks of dynamic local health systems. On the other hand, there is the orthodox tradition of public services as philanthropy, where a 'normative consensus' provides the motivation and care and corporacy go hand in hand (Etzioni 1971). In this model the public services were contrasted with private companies, divided into their specialist functions and driven by the calculative commitment of increasing profits and the shareholders' returns; or a voluntary organization where people come together more loosely with less formal roles in an association of similar interests and like minds (Table 5.1). Such a theoretical framework never really did justice to, for example, the massive political and small business dimensions of the NHS. It certainly does not do so now.

Nevertheless, regardless of their relevance, both conceptual models continue to be used, especially in official documentation. If not mental sloth, this does seem to be a

Table 5.1. Characteristics of pre-1990 organizations

	Purpose	Process	Form
Private	Profit	Calculative Commitment	Company
Public	Service	Normative Integration	Bureaucracy
Voluntary	Membership	Affective Affiliation	Association

[based on Etzioni (1971)]

form of intellectual inertia. Figure 5.1, for example, is taken from *The New NHS: Modern, Dependable* white paper (Secretary of State for Health 1997, p21). It depicts the future post-1997 organization, conventionally in structural terms, as a new type of hierarchy. A map showing the networks, coalitions and alliances in sociogram style would be more suitable and certainly more accurate in describing the NHS nationwide. But we have found people in the NHS often too tired, or even too fearful, to engage critically and constructively with contemporary organizational developments. It seems almost better to live with an illusion: the external public still needs to feel secure about the continuity of the NHS as an organization however fluid its internal realities may be. On the inside this myth of continuity is sharply at odds with the change agenda of a millennium workforce wanting the mobility and flexibility that goes with today's lifestyles, but not with the lifelong professions and practices around which the NHS was built. This internal agenda simply further fuels the pressure for continuous organizational uncertainty (Bell 1999).

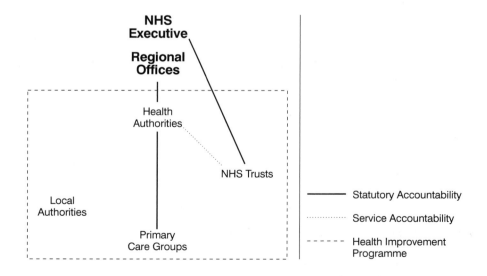

Fig. 5.1. New NHS accountabilities (Secretary of State for Health 1997, p21)

(Dis)integrated diversity in practice

Nevertheless, central statements often continue to assume consensus, taking support and success for granted. The increasingly pluralistic nature of the UK health system is skimmed over, with the new range of both positive and negative definitions of health (Aggleton 1990) reflected in the emerging variety of healthcare agencies. In primary care alone there are now health centres, surgeries, resource centres, community care units, healthy living centres, Healthcall companies, health parks, complementary medicine and pastoral care centres and intermediate care facilities – which is a list in double figures of sites where GPs can (usually) still be counted as the main contributors. The number would easily double if nurse-led schemes were added. Health means different things in different places and so too now does its organization. The new NHS emphasis is on restoring effective 'strategic coordination' through such novel national organizations as the National Institute for Clinical Excellence (NICE) and by means of robust national standards to reinforce its values. 'Fragmentation' is, therefore, regarded as the enemy (Secretary of State for Health 1997, pp10–14). But while this is a target that can be applied legitimately to service delivery, and the patient experience of this, if 'fragmentation' includes organizational developments in its aim, the rich potential of the latter for enhancing relationships and thence health itself – however defined – will be sorely neglected. Diversity of organizations and services is an absolutely essential part of primary healthcare when its principles of participation and intersectoral collaboration are put into practice (Macdonald 1992, pp85–123, Starfield 1992). This is a very hard lesson for the NHS and its political masters to learn. They may not in the end be willing to do so.

Clearly more attention needs to be given to the nature of the contemporary organization, especially at local levels. Perhaps the detailed guidance on *Developing Primary Care Groups* (NHS Executive 1998 pp6–7) illustrates this shortfall best. The functions are crystal clear:

▶ to improve the health and address the health inequalities of local communities

▶ to develop integrated primary and community care services of consistent quality

▶ to commission effective secondary care with shorter waiting periods

But the organizational means are not. The overall aim is fulsome:

> 'to modernize the NHS so that it is fast and convenient, guarantees uniformly high standards, integrates services around the needs of patients not institutions and tackles the causes of ill health as well as illness and disability'.
>
> (NHS Executive 1998 para 1)

The organizational support for this is listed as 'providing the resources required', 'the use of modern technology' and a 'progressive employer' approach – all at national level. The personal, social and behavioural requirements of organizational development are scarcely referred to at all and certainly not in respect of primary care groups (PCGs). The 1998 health service circular on PCG development devotes 65 pages to the organizational requirements. Of these 57 are on the subjects of accountability, budgets and structures (NHS Executive 1998). PCG development as health and healthcare organizations is assumed. The practice of local organization is not a subject for central attention. The theory is there, at national level. At this level it can be applied to organizational development and that it would appear is enough, at least for the time being.

The relational dividend

Legacy of change

Yet the assumption that all will be well with organizational development is being (mis)placed at the level where it can be least confidently guaranteed. This is the level where, between 1990 and 1996, over 400 statutory NHS organizations were terminated. Some in effect actually disappeared twice, eg family practitioner committees and family health services authorities. This trend has continued since the 1997 general election. In Scotland there are no longer any NHS community health services trusts; there are now only two worthy of the title left in Wales. In Northern Ireland the centrally favoured option for 2001 is the dissolution of the four health boards. Over 3000 fundholding units have disappeared across the UK.

What does all this mean for the local experience? If you worked in Bath, for example, between 1994 and the end of 1998 you would have been accountable to no fewer than four NHS regional bodies: almost one a year in terms of turnover. In the London area between 1991 and 2001 there is now the real prospect of a four-fold reduction in the number of health authorities within the decade. This is not so much organizational change as organizational collapse, and certainly this description captures accurately the feelings of many local NHS participants who have engaged with the Relational Health Care (RHC) project during the 1996–1999 period. The turnover in organizations has been interesting if you have been in a position to observe; exciting if you have been a beneficiary in terms of promotion or pecuniary reward; but too often disappointing or even devastating if you have been 'streamlined', labelled as 'excess bureaucracy' or 'downsized'. The 1990s NHS has left many organizations and many more individuals on the defensive.

Organizational suicide

In terms of forming PCGs or taking forward, for example, inter-NHS trust collaborative ventures, this means that the relationships required have a difficult starting point. The dilemma this general malaise brings with it is nicely captured in Figure 5.2.

This is a Dutch cartoon. It became popular with the directors of some local hospitals in the Netherlands when the merger of public 'sickness funds' with private health insurance companies was allowed by the Dutch government in the mid-1990s. The aim was to reduce costs, improve efficiency and tackle expensive secondary care providers. The principal targets were hospitals. The directors knew that some could be expected to close, but only after they had kept the healthcare show on the road while the insurance agencies were distracted by the messy process of mergers. Indeed, during this phase, a fair amount of handholding was called for by the new 'purchasers' from the

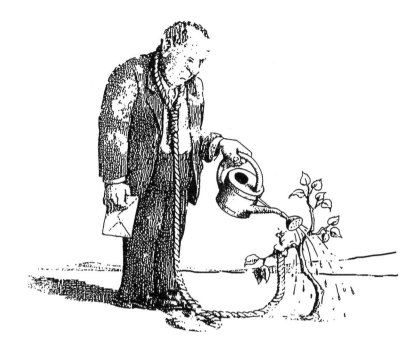

Figure 5.2 Self-destructing NHS?

traditional 'providers'. The directors were right. Several hospitals did close, or became incorporated into larger units, including in areas like Rotterdam where the service demand pressures on them were greatest during the period when the new commissioning arrangements were becoming established.

Back in the UK we were not surprised when a couple of sets of acute services NHS trust board members identified with this cartoon. We were surprised, however, when it became clear that so did everybody else. Health authority managers, nurses, GPs and even GP fundholders all reacted in the same way. They all saw in themselves the man with the noose around his neck. All felt as if they were being set up to be strangled.

Fluid stability

It was only in July 1997, just after the general election and Labour's proclamation of a 'new NHS' in the Queen's Speech, that somebody suggested simply taking the noose off, by freeing one hand and lifting it over his head. The timing may have been a coincidence but it pointed to a potentially different set of relationships between the central and local boundaries of the NHS in the future, in which organizations could have greater control over their own survival and health.

This is the relational dividend. For those responsible for formulating policy there is the prize of being able to plan delivery through relationships rather than through conventional organizational units. The former offer a prospect of greater permanence, stronger commitment and wider participation. In short they are a basis for policies that last – provided the people last too.

For those responsible for delivering health services the relational dividend offers the challenge and freedom to create contemporary organizations, without structural prescription. Implementation can take greater account of the human dimension and local circumstances. The noose can be discarded.

Contemporary organizations

But this is not yet how the organization of the new NHS feels. Especially at the local level, the majority remain suspicious of central intent. Being able to convert heroic rhetoric about partnerships into daily working processes remains an elusive ideal when the organizational models that might be able to achieve this conversion are still either little understood or applied. As we noted above, even in academic circles the pace of organizational change has outstripped research capacity. A new theory of organization is still required, especially for the public services sector.

In the absence of this theory, however, trends and concepts are emerging; which is where, as one of the most vivid expressions of these new ideas, PCGs fit in. 'What sort of organization do we want to be?' is a basic question all leaders of new primary care organizations are asking themselves. Over the past two years we have found that for those looking to create enterprises which strengthen local relationships three simple ideas are proving helpful. Each ensures that the PCG releases itself from the practice-based insularity which has generally characterized primary care in the UK in the past. Each term is entering common parlance. Together the concepts and models expressed through these terms may be the basis for integrating tomorrow's organizational theory and practice.

Virtual organizations

The first and most popular phrase is that of the 'virtual organization'. Its features are a sense of belonging for participants beyond their host employer and its physical base, overarching and simply stated strategic aims and widespread personal identification with these. British Airways and Virgin are the most commonly cited examples of 'virtual organizations'; but the NHS itself is assuming some of the traits. Certainly when working, for example, with GPs in emerging PCGs in Cornwall and Somerset, where decentralization is everything, it can easily seem like the 'New NHS' means little more than a popular brand name. The local patch is everything. Their identification with the corporate identity is far less say than that of 'Air Miles' staff with British Airways.

PCGs are certainly 'virtual organizations'. Table 5.2 sets out the roles and responsibilities of PCGs as summarized in the original 'New NHS' policy statements. This indicates clearly that at Levels 1 and 2, PCGs are not discrete, formal organizations. At Level 2, for example, they are subcommittees of a health authority but operate 'as if' they are something more: representing a full cross-section of primary care professionals; operating to clinical governance standards and overseeing financial allocations and prescribing performance. Virtually all aspects of extended primary care fall within their remit.

Table 5.2. Roles and responsibilities of PCGs (Secretary of State for Health 1997)

Level	Role and responsibilities
1	As a minimum to act in support of the health authority in commissioning care for the district population, acting in an advisory capacity
2	To take devolved responsibility for managing the budget for healthcare in their PCG area, acting as a committee of the health authority
3	As a PCT to become established as a free-standing body accountable to the health authority for the commissioning of healthcare
4	As for Level 3 but with additional responsibility for the provision of community health services to the population in the PCG area

Even at Level 4, the 'virtual organization' analogy applies. When we worked with the Local Health Care Cooperative in St Andrews, for example, this was very evident. The GPs remained independent contractors and the practice nurses were still employed by them; but both were also very much part of the wider NHS primary care trust (PCT). It was as participants in the latter, for example, that they were planning combined health and social care emergency facilities; wanted to lobby the new Scottish Assembly in Edinburgh for additional funding; and planned to negotiate the assumption of additional commissioning duties from 1999/2000 with the trust chief executive and other local healthcare cooperatives.

As this example from their Scottish counterparts illustrates, the recognition of themselves as 'virtual organizations' can help liberate PCGs. In relational terms it releases a range of primary care professionals from the restrictions of their traditional pecking orders, as well as more prosaically from the constraints of the job description. The GP pays the practice nurse, but it is the NHS which funds the practice. The 'virtual organization' concept allows both these relationships to operate effectively. In Reading, Thurrock and Aldershot, for example, we have seen the contribution of health visitors to health needs assessment actually restored and reaffirmed by local PCGs, as the latter have begun to address their new NHS responsibilities for promoting public health. The 'virtual organization' is not without its perils especially in terms of possible split loyalties. It does mean, however, that the organizational development of primary care is responding to PCGs' new strategic roles, while sustaining its operational strengths. It also means that those in primary care can take the relationship skills and sensitivities which are at the very heart of their practice into a much wider range of community forums and networks. Already in other parts of the healthcare environment the 'virtual organization' idea holds sway. In research the Cochrane Centre operates to this model. In training one of the Relationship Foundation's recent partners, Capita Business Services Limited, deploys a wide range of formal and informal associates just as if they were part of a single organization. If research and training can operate on a relationships basis then surely the omens are encouraging for the 'new' primary care.

Stakeholder organizations

If the concept of 'virtual organization' is an important new psychological resource for PCGs and their internal staff, that of the 'stakeholder organization' is, perhaps, of more tangible and visible benefit. In the first instance it applies to the resource base of the organization and either its consolidation or extension. The 'stakeholder organization' comprises a new mix of finance, capital and personnel drawn from across the conventional public and private sectors; and includes voluntary or commercial contributions. As a result the range of accountabilities increases but rather than creating a source of tension this is seen as a means of ensuring powerful stakeholders have a real incentive in collaborating with others to achieve overall corporate success. In this organizational context sound relationships are vital. Past barriers between separate sectors can no longer be tolerated. This, of course, is the kind of thinking that has gone into the government's policy for new action zones, with those for both health and education focusing on deprived areas where the intersectoral collaboration principle pivotal to modern primary healthcare (Duggan 1995, McDonald 1992, p109) has been little practised but is most needed. It is also the kind of thinking that has resulted in the NHS from the new Labour government's current examination of the implications of the Private Finance Initiative (PFI) and their application of methods of communication in pursuit of "modernised public services". Developments in information technology have perhaps been the most influential and partisan factors in the growing literature on 'stakeholder organizations' (eg Wheeler and Sillanpää 1997).

The extent to which PCGs are emerging as 'stakeholder organizations' has been understated. The new mixed economy of frontline care does not always seem to sit so comfortably with ministerial assertions that the traditional public NHS is being restored, albeit in 'modernized' mode (Prime Minister's speech at the Health Conference, Birmingham, 13 April 1999). In November 1998, as part of the action research project addressing the relationship between public health and new primary care organizations (see p42–54), we met with 25 colleagues drawn from local PCGs and health authorities. The following districts were represented: West Pennine, Leeds, Barking and Havering, Southampton and South West Hampshire, West Hertfordshire and Nottinghamshire. By the end of the day the extent to which PCGs already embraced a wide range of different stakeholders was apparent. Table 5.3 was the result. This list is something of a revelation for both resource and relationships management. In some areas the potential for both is enormous.

One of the PCGs on the edge of the New Forest viewed the local allotment society as a key relational resource in its south coast site. Some of the GPs were trustees of the society which had a sizeable legacy of land sales proceeds and covenants. This was one kind of joint venture perhaps requiring charitable foundation status. Others, of a different order, were with the Royal Bank of Scotland in Fife, a London commodities

Table 5.3. PCGs' organizational status

(a) Health authority subcommittee (public)
(b) Prospective NHS trust (with access to PFI)
(c) Legal partnership (independent)
(d) (Not-for-profit) Limited company (private)
(e) Joint venture (commercial)
(f) Charitable foundation (voluntary)
(g) Local patients' association (community)

(Meads et al 1999)

broker and social entrepreneur in south London and Leicestershire where either trust status (for PFIs) or the use of fundholders' not-for-profit companies could be used to take joint stakes in developing GP hospitals.

The 'stakeholder organization' has obvious business overtones. Its application in respect of PCGs is compelling the new NHS to revisit its long-held assumptions about the private sector and business ethics. These assumptions have contained some crude stereotypes about commercial self-interest. With PCGs now charged with a responsibility for public health that can only be achieved by productive relationships across the public and independent sectors, attitudes must change. The organizational frameworks required are those that can enable this to happen. Devlin's (1998) recent study of the modern relationship between primary healthcare services and the private sector illustrates this. Her empirically-based criteria for partnership accordingly include some conventional public values (eg joint objectives), but also some in terms of agreed exit and risk-sharing strategies that would previously have been unacceptable both to the political and professionals powers of the old NHS institution (Table 5.4).

Table 5.4. Reasons partnerships work

▶ Individual and joint objectives coincide
▶ Reciprocity becomes the motivating force
▶ Process is managed with internal review milestones and external success markers
▶ Common 'enemy' remains to the fore
▶ Damage limitation exit strategy held in reserve

[based on Devlin (1998), p68]

Community organizations

A step beyond the 'stakeholder organization' is that of the 'community organization'. This emerging organizational concept is now helping to strengthen the relationships base of the new NHS. For PCGs we have seen it used most either where the local leadership is most committed to achieving Level 4 status as the organizational basis for combining health and social services (eg Oldham, East Southampton, Daventry) or where the full involvement of public representatives is regarded as paramount to the future success of local health groups (eg in the south Wales districts of Bro Taf and Ichyd Morgannyg). These two strands of local development come together in the concept and its significance. 'Community organization' denotes not only an organization whose first relationship is to its local community, but also an organization which is in itself a community.

In this second sense the 'community organization' embraces a new and wider range of both people and functions. Figure 5.3, as used by the local health groups in Gwent, illustrates this comprehensive variety of tasks. More important for relationships, however, is the 'community organization' of people. In this model the sense of belonging moves on from stakeholding to a genuine sense of ownership. Participants can become members and the membership may include managers, professionals, patients and the public. This is the route for PCGs to travel if they wish to approach their clients as enrolled members, sharing in decisions about service priorities, rather than merely as registered patients receiving clinically determined treatments. It is a

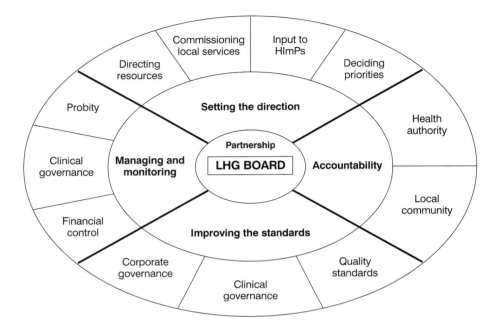

Figure 5.3. Overview of local health group board role

route on which we have witnessed the first steps taken by GPs in, for example, Winchester, Derby and Lyme Regis – in other words right across the country.

Community organization and community development used to be concepts applied to describe two contrasting approaches to organizational development at local level (Thomas 1976). Community development was the non-directive, bottom-up approach. It produced pressure groups, neighbourhood councils, parents' associations and the like. The form reflected the purpose. The skill in organizational development was in harnessing the energy of informal relationships. Community organization, on the other hand, was about formal relationships. The organizational development process was through public appointments and electoral systems. A local authority could be a community organization; so could an Anglican church. The challenge for PCGs is to see whether or not they can harness the strengths of both these approaches. If they can, the strength of their formal and informal relationships' infrastructure will give them a local legitimacy the NHS has never before experienced in its 50-year history.

Organizational learning

If the 'virtual', 'stakeholder' and 'community' organizations are all still very much embryonic concepts, then that of the 'learning organization' is now much more firmly established. The research- and consultancy-based publications of Handy (1985) and

Senge (1990) have been the chief sources of this model and it has been recently augmented by a number of contemporary health management thinkers (eg Iles 1997). Senge (1990, p14) defined the learning organization first as 'an organization that is continually expanding its capacity to create its future'.

Personal mastery or central control?

This capacity is based on a new integration of a series of modern sources of knowledge, including systems thinking, mental modelling (or scenario planning) and what Senge (1990, p7) terms 'personal mastery': the 'cornerstone' and 'spiritual foundation' of the learning organization. Together these disciplines are required as the source of innovation which provides the competitive edge for survival in today's increasingly complex environment. Together they ensure the learning organization is in a constant dynamic exchange with this environment. As a result it is a key source of its continuous changes. For individuals this means the prospect of developing what Handy termed 'career portfolios'.

Much of the new NHS as a national organization is very much in this mode: taking whole systems approaches in, for example, its approach to quality or IT, setting out the shared vision of *Modernising Health and Social Services* (Department of Health and Social Services 1999), and looking quite consciously beyond the millennium to 2030 in terms of its models for future hospitals and their configuration. For primary care this national 'learning organization' approach has meant turning policy on its head in terms of its basic perspectives. We are witnessing 'NHS-led primary care'. The centre is setting the direction. The previous government's banner headline was the other way around. 'A primary care-led NHS' (NHS Executive 1994), meant not just simply a further range of GP fundholders with extended purchasing responsibilities, but also a sense of trust in real delegation of power to local professionals in terms of setting the direction (of diversity) for the modern NHS, through local professionals rather than politicians' relationships with the public'.

This analysis suggests, accordingly, that in terms of the 'learning organization' theoretical model, the post-1997 NHS may score less highly on Senge's disciplines of 'personal mastery' and 'team learning' than its predecessor. The conditions for genuine dialogue in 'thinking together' about the significance of the changing organizational environment, and the space continually to retain and adopt a shared vision which stands the test of objectivity to give individuals a sense of their 'personal mastery' (Senge 1990, pp7–11), are both less than they were. Local individuals have less license in both these areas. The first six items on the agendas of most of the PCG meetings we have attended are centrally determined. The first comprehensive assessment of health improvement programmes (HImPs) across London health districts in 1998/1999 (NHS Executive London Regional Office 1999) found that national priorities were invariably included but local variations, whether from PCGs or elsewhere, were now relatively few and far between and clearly less evident than in past fundholders' plans. General practices had been much more effective in advocating for their particular concerns than they were in collaborating to agree joint priorities. Accordingly, the new NHS as a learning organization is much more apparent in its central than its local components and the former are not of themselves sufficient yet to suggest that a national learning

Table 5.5. Future criteria for organizational development of primary care organizations

A *Partnership:*
► Inter-professional
► Intersectoral
► Demonstrable community involvement
► Enrolled patients
► Healthcare programmes oriented
► Care management
► Maximized income sources
► Role flexibility
► Participative culture
► Systemic quality
► Equitable benefits

B *Decentralization*
► Effective teamwork processes and structures
► Combinations of informal and formal carers
► Coherent priority-setting processes
► Increased resource management responsibilities
► Demonstrable accountability systems – public and professional
► Support of elected, appointed and user representatives
► Compliance with NHS strategies and values
► Incorporation in district Health Investment Programmes
► Effective local strategic alliances within and beyond NHS

organization is emerging. Senge's two key relationally-oriented disciplines – team learning and personal mastery – will require considerable future attention if the full model is to apply.

Partnership and decentralization

This will mean an openness to organizational learning. Table 5.5 details the criteria for effective organizational development that PCGs and their successors are expected to meet. The requirements for 'partnership' are wide ranging, novel and immensely challenging. Genuine participation, for example, has been anathema to much of general practice. Its essentially individualistic if not egotistic orientation in the past indicates the extent to which broad-based approaches to local communities, systems and other and new kinds of professions will be a journey across new territory. The ride is bound to be bumpy, with breakdowns part of the package.

The 'decentralization' list is equally daunting. Decisions taken in parliament 10 years ago will now be taken in primary care. Erratically but inexorably public health and primary care are fusing. The organizational criteria mean that clinical and financial responsibilities are being taken as one.

The organizational learning requirements at the local level are immense and for PCGs in particular will not simply just happen. They will only happen if we look outwards as well as inwards. The learning organization is all about the interests of your own organization. Organizational learning is broader. It represents the collective self-interest. Its essence is learning what is best for organizations *in toto*, at all levels: local, central and intermediate, and for all their relationships: lateral, vertical and diagonal. This means the tenacious, but inevitably sometimes tentative, exploration together of such new relationship-oriented organizational ideas as the 'virtual', 'stakeholder' and 'community' organizations in order to find a contemporary practice and theory that fits together and can feed future policy. The dividend for health and healthcare relationships of a successful search will be substantial and this is one search where the Internet, for once, will not be of much use. As has recently been pointed out 'knowledge-driven' organizations in the private sector could very easily jeopardize the survival of the traditional 'people businesses' such as design and advertising (Bell 1999). The search in the public sector for the kinds of healthcare organization we now need begins and ends with ourselves.

Summary

The pace of change in the practice of organizations has outstripped organizational theory. New concepts are required, especially at local levels in primary care. Here the requirements for partnerships are such that future organizational relationships will have to be both more numerous and more productive. The ideas involved in 'virtual', 'stakeholder' and 'community' organizations are proving helpful, especially in primary care, in regenerating the new NHS.

References

Aggleton P (1990). *Health*. London: Routledge: Ch 1.
Bell M (1999). The knowledge revolution. In: *Resource*. London: Capita: 14–15.
Department of Health (1999). *Modernising Health and Social Services: Developing the Workforce,* HSC 1999/111, LAC (99)18. Leeds: NHS Executive, Leeds.
Devlin M (1998). *Primary Health Care and the Private Sector*. Oxford: Radcliffe Medical Press.
Duggan M (1995). *Primary Health Care: A Prognosis*. London: IPPR.
Etzioni A (1971). *A Comparative Analysis of Complex Organisations*. New York: Free Press.
Handy C (1985). *Understanding Organisations*. Harmondsworth: Penguin.
Iles V (1997). *Really Managing Health Care*. Buckingham: Open University Press.
Macdonald J (1992). *Primary Health Care: Medicine in its Place*. London: Earthscan.
Meads G, Killoran A, Ashcroft J, Cornish Y (1999). *Mixing Oil and Water*. London: HEA Publications: 30.
NHS Executive (1994). *Developing NHS Purchasing and GP Fundholding: Towards a Primary Care-Led NHS,* EL (94) 79. Leeds: Department of Health.
NHS Executive (1998). *The New NHS: Modern and Dependable: Developing Primary Care Groups*, HSC 1998/139. Leeds: Department of Health.
NHS Executive London Regional Office (1999). *London's Health Improvement Programmes. Findings from the First Phase of Development 1998/99*. London: NHS Executive.
Secretary of State for Health (1997). *The New NHS: Modern, Dependable*, Cm 3807. London: HMSO.
Starfield B (1992). *Primary Care: Concept, Policy and Evaluation*. Oxford: Oxford University Press: Ch 1.
Senge P (1990). *The Fifth Discipline. The Art and Science of Learning Organisation*. London: Century.
Thomas D (1976). *Organising for Social Change: A Study in the Theory and Practice of Community Work*. London: Allen and Unwin.
Weber M. (translated by Henderson AM and Talcott Parsons) (1947). *The Theory of Social and Economic Organisation*. Illinois: Free Press of Glencoe: 132–4.
Wheeler D and Sillanpää M (1997). *The Stakeholder Corporation*. London: Pitman Publishing.

6
Delivery

'If one falls down, his friend can help him up.
But pity the man who falls and has no-one to help him up!'
(Ecclesiastes 4: 10)

Core function and main concern

The issue of delivering relational healthcare raises many questions about who delivers what, to whom and how. The basic thesis of this project has been that there is a relational dimension to health which has too often been neglected; and that healthcare requires collaborative relationships among those involved in provision and caring relationships with patients. This is not intended to imply that patients should not be collaborative partners in their own healthcare, that 'caring' provides a comprehensive account of appropriate therapeutic relationships, or that the concern for care is confined to patients – it should apply to staff as well.

This thesis, rather baldly stated, has a number of important implications. If relationships and social support are an important aspect of health, then any attempts to 'seek a healthier nation' should include a concern for the relational fabric of society. If 'caring' is important for the wellbeing of patients, then relationships with patients and working practices must enable caring to take place. If effective delivery requires collaboration between individuals, professions and organizations, then the obstacles to such collaboration must be overcome.

Getting this right is important because the delivery of healthcare and improved health is the core function of the health service. It is the litmus test against which the impact of policy, resources, strategy, organizational change and professional development must be tested. In practice delivery may not always feel like the core function. For those involved in the frontline of delivery it can seem as though their activity adjusts to support other functions, such as resource management, rather than defining their purpose. There is also always the danger that an organization, or elements of its activity, becomes self-serving. This may reflect personal, professional or organizational interests within or outside the NHS. This is illustrated by the reforms of the early 1990s which Klein (1995) argues were more about making the NHS itself, rather than the government, accountable for any problems in delivery than directly addressing problems in the delivery of healthcare. It is therefore no surprise that delivery (however this function is defined) is often the focal point of many concerns about the health service.

The definition of what delivery should constitute remains hotly debated, with competing health ideologies and models of therapeutic relationships typically being to the fore. The ripples of disagreement spread out through all the other functions and may become manifest in disagreements over policy, strategy, resource allocations, the kinds of organization most suitable for delivery, the development needed to support it or definitions of quality. In practice, during the Relational Health Care (RHC), project we have found greater consensus than these debates might imply, although this has frequently been masked by the persistence of stereotyped views about other health professionals' beliefs and significant gaps between espoused and expressed values. The latter is a consequence of a wide range of practical and systemic constraints on delivery.

Another feature of delivery as a function is that it is of central importance yet cannot be directly controlled. It can be influenced, constrained, fostered or undermined, but in the end healthcare (and much health improvement) is delivered by individuals, alone or in teams. The new NHS sees delivery as being, ultimately, a professional issue, but seeks to influence delivery by shaping the context and impact of other functions. A stronger focus on public health strategy will, for example, influence what is delivered, in turn influencing who is involved in the process and the structures and systems to support it. New organizations are created to 'deliver the agenda' [primary care groups (PCGs)], as well as to monitor and advise that delivery [eg the National Institute for Clinical Excellence (NICE) and the Commission for Health Improvement]. Expectations of cultural change are set out in terms of the 'duty of partnership' or the accessibility of a modernized service. But within this changing context delivery remains the responsibility of the medical professions:

> *'local doctors and nurses who are in the best position to know what patients need will be in the driving seat of shaping services.'*
>
> (Secretary of State for Health 1997)

For the professions part of this responsibility has been (on behalf of both patients and their own interest) to question the impact of changes (or failure to change) on the delivery of healthcare. It is this concern which prompted the start of the RHC project. Yet delivery has not, directly, been a major focus of much of the project. We have addressed, to varying extents, the other core functions but have not, for example, worked with patients and providers to improve service delivery. In this we have in part followed the agenda of the new NHS. As the project moves more firmly into a review phase, looking at the impact of the changing relational environment on the delivery of healthcare will become more important.

Thus the project will both start and end with a focus on delivery, the importance of which was evident in our initial consultations. There was an almost daily litany of inadequate relationships (with doctors at times resenting managerial intrusion into the sanctum of professional therapeutic relationships); frustration about waiting times and consequent delayed diagnosis and treatment, the embarrassment of cancelled opera-tions and concerns about the fragmentation of care – both between specialisms within the acute sector and throughout the health economy. There was a combination of personal, clinical and professional concerns. For many doctors there appeared to be a profound sense of loss: constraints on their ability to care and loss of relationships with patients and colleagues, values or vocation.

It is worth attempting to recapture something of the mood of a few years ago; press cuttings provide one useful (if unscientific) indicator. Looking back at those of 1995 we find morale was being described as in crisis: the BMA stating that a quarter of junior doctors have become so disenchanted with the health service that they are no longer working in medicine (*The Independent* 4 July 1995), and that they are less likely to view medicine as a vocation than their elders: among doctors over 55, one in six viewed medicine as a vocation compared with one in 100 among those under 30 (BMA survey of 800 members quoted in *The Times* 15 December 95). A survey in *Doctor* magazine reports that two-thirds of GPs who responded wanted to leave the NHS (quoted in *Financial Times* 16 May 95) while the BMA reports that the number of GPs taking early retirement has increased by 50% over the last decade (*Financial Times* 29 September 95). Nurses appear unhappy too, with an RCN survey reporting that four in 10 would leave the profession if they could (*The Daily Telegraph* 4 December 95). Books such as Bruggen's (1997) *Who Cares* capture this mood with what Dr Macara (then chairman of the BMA) describes as 'a cathartic testimony of health professionals and managers caught up in the dehumanising culture change in the NHS'.

Another striking feature of the consultations at the start of the project was the diversity of views and strengths of stereotypes revealing divisions within and between professions. There were many who welcomed changes in healthcare delivery, but issues such as fundholding and the introduction of the internal market had divided professions. The background of difficult interprofessional relationships was felt to hinder attempts to address concerns about healthcare delivery. In the course of our initial consultation period doctors were criticized for their lack of commitment to public health, disinterest in effective management and obstruction of change. Managers were still frequently disparaged as grey-suited bean-counters with no real commitment to patients or the core values of the NHS. Nurses' aspirations and skills were too readily dismissed.

The delivery of healthcare can become a battleground. It may be ideological – over different definitions of health; it may be over resources; or over professional roles. It can result in competing claims for advocacy with, for example, both medical professions and government claiming to be advocates of patients' interests against the other. The delivery of health can also be a unifying function. The shared concern to do better for patients can be a powerful engine for change. Many RHC project participants have found the changing face of primary care a liberating and exciting experience, with the opportunity to forge new partnerships in healthcare delivery leading to tangible benefits for patients. Yet there are others for whom the concerns of four years ago ring just as powerfully today. Until lasting improvements in the delivery of improved health and healthcare can be shown the new NHS will remain on trial.

Relational health

Definitions of health and models of healthcare relationships have been the subject of much academic debate: this has focused on such issues as patient-centred care (eg

Fulford *et al* 1996), healthcare partnerships (eg Farrell and Gilbert 1996), philosophies of nursing (eg Bradshaw 1994) or collaborative relationships (eg Hudson 1998). Our objective is rather more modest: to illustrate some of the practical expressions of these issues encountered in our work and to consider how a more supportive environment for the delivery of relational healthcare might be created.

The issue of the definition of health has come to the fore in the RHC project in two ways. The first was the concerns of the clinicians who encouraged the start of the project. For these doctors medicine was a calling, a vocation. A major concern was how to combine clinical excellence with care for the whole person. For some this focused on the issue of how concerns for spiritual and physical (or mental) health could be better integrated. For others it was the recognition that as individuals, and as a service, they were ill-equipped to deal with the wide range of non-medical problems with which patients came to them (either as the underlying causes of medical symptoms or as the presenting issue itself). They felt it was increasingly difficult to match a broad account of human wellbeing with the services they were able to provide. One aspect of the problem was philosophical and ethical: the definition of health and the healthcare values that should underpin the health service. Another was the practicalities of constrained relationships with patients and other healthcare professions which hindered the integration of care and the balance of 'caring' and 'curing'. Time, and flexibility in the use of time under the scrutiny of performance management, was a particular concern here.

The second angle on this issue has been the importance of public health in health policy and strategy. During the RHC project we have repeatedly encountered the belief that doctors are not interested in public health (expressed, for example, by some GPs about their colleagues or by senior health authority staff). This has not been the reality for the great majority of doctors (admittedly often from 'leading-edge' primary care sites) who have participated in RHC projects. The missed opportunities as a result were vividly illustrated in the professional depression of a public health manager in a North Western health authority who stated that 99% of GPs were not interested in public health, unaware that a lead GP (in the same workshop) was a more passionate advocate of public health than many of the directors of public health we have encountered. In a health strategy simulation looking at the potential for PCGs to improve public health (see p51–54) a group of health authority staff based their strategy on the assumption that GPs would, by and large, be working with a narrow medical view of health.

There is, however, sufficient truth in the continuing influence of a narrow medical model of health for such views to persist. This model has been used with a variety of meanings (Macklin 1973). The model is steeped in the scientific tradition of medicine, tends to see health as 'functional normality' (Boorse 1981) and focuses on biological explanations of ill health. As a comprehensive model of health it may not represent the beliefs of many health professionals, but continues to be evident in their practice, as shaped by many factors such as professional training, organizational structures or commissioning processes. A number of criticisms are ranged against this model (eg Engel 1981, Guttmacher 1979, Jubilee Centre 1998, Laura and Heaney 1990, Sharkey 1992). It is criticized for being reductionist, both in terms of not treating the whole person and in ignoring the wider social and environmental determinants of health. It may undermine the unity of the person so that psychological, spiritual and social dimensions of health are not treated in an integrated way. This may lead to ineffective treatment which does not deal with the root causes of or fails to prevent ill health, or which is experienced as depersonalized and dehumanizing. It focuses on treatment by skilled professionals and may alienate the patient (and carers) from the healing process. The persistent prevalence of some forms of ill health [eg coronary heart disease (CHD) or cancer] and the re-emergence of diseases such as tuberculosis also point to the limits of a purely medical model of health.

Broader definitions of health such as that of the World Health Organization ('Health is a state of complete physical, mental and social wellbeing and not merely the absence of disease or infirmity') may be accepted in theory but are not always expressed in practice. Holistic definitions of health are not particularly helpful in defining or circumscribing the roles of health professionals. In practice it may at times be more helpful to accept a narrower definition of health, but set within the context of a broader vision of human wellbeing and an integrated understanding of the person which recognizes the potential interplay of physical, mental, social and spiritual states. There will, however, always be the danger that this broader context is neglected or its achievement undermined by, for example, the nature of professional training, interprofessional and interorganizational relationships, care practices and the organizational structures and systems of the NHS.

The concept of relational health can aid integration. Learning to see and think about individuals in their relational context may point both to such health-inhibiting factors as lack of social support as well as the work of other agencies and professions that are seeking to promote the patient's wellbeing. Seeing the broader social, economic and environmental determinants of health in relational terms helps avoid seeing them purely as remote impersonal forces. They are consequences of how individuals, communities, organizations and the state interrelate.

The issue is not just one of patient satisfaction but of demonstrable medical benefits. The link between relationships and health is complex, with many factors in play. Three important links are the impact of relationships on healthy (or unhealthy) behaviours, on stress and the tolerance of stress, and on care and social support. These links are, at least in part, the probable explanation for the broad statistical links between marital status and health which have been established for some time (eg Lynch 1977). Death rates for CHD, cancer of the digestive organs and vascular lesions are all lower for married men and women than for those who are divorced, widowed or single. The health benefits of marriage are much greater for men than for women. More work is needed to unravel the many factors and to establish the relative significance of relationships as a health-promoting or -inhibiting factor. There is, however, sufficient evidence to suggest that its importance may be underestimated and that current public health strategies are limited in their capacity to address these issues. The evidence below is not a comprehensive review, but serves to illustrate some of the issues to be addressed.

Good relationships have health benefits, but dysfunctional or no relationships can contribute to ill health. The effects of stress, for example, are widespread, being linked to increased vulnerability to viral infections, atherosclerosis, onset of diabetes, asthma and ulceration of the gastrointestinal tract (McEwen and Stellar 1993, Kennedy *et al*

1988). Dysfunctional relationships, at home or at work, can be major causes of stress. Conversely supportive relationships can aid management of stress. In the workplace strong support from co-workers and supervisors results in no significant link between workplace stress and health (Caplan *et al* 1975). Rosengren *et al* (1993) reported that Swedish men who had 'a dependable web of intimacy' showed no link between high stress levels and death rate. This contrasts with an overall three-fold increase in the death rate for those men who did not have this 'web' and reported being under intense emotional stress.

Goleman (1995) summarizes some of the studies on CHD, one of the national priorities for public health. It may be affected by emotional state, particularly anger (Ironson 1992, Mittleman 1994) or anxiety (Thoreson 1990). Death rates are reduced by social support (Berkman *et al* 1992). This may be through more positive emotional support, better compliance with medical advice, practical care or healthier lifestyles. There are important implications here for medical practice. The *National Service Framework for Coronary Heart Disease* (Department of Health 1998), for example, is strong on interagency working, but is silent on how relational health could contribute to health improvement in this area.

It also raises questions about what a healthier nation might look like. There are many symptoms of increasing relational pressure, not just through such obvious headline figures as high divorce rates. Many factors put relationships under pressure (Baker 1996): patterns of work, mobility affecting the extended family, urban design and town planning, or the impact of technology. Every age and every society faces its own different set of pressures on relationships. They do not determine our behaviour, but will often influence it. Relationship trends are complex phenomena and in assessing the impact of changes there are usually debits and credits, neither of which may be easily quantifiable, to be considered. These are not uncontrollable forces: in many cases they are issues on which we can, or could have, choice or at a minimum where the relational consequences can be better managed. If we are committed to seeking a healthier nation we neglect its relational health at our peril.

Relational care

The concerns of many project participants about caring are summarized in Kitson's (1996) plea from a nurse's perspective on patient-centred care:

> *'Just having time to talk or be with a patient is becoming increasingly difficult in today's cost-conscious healthcare system. What will happen if nurses and doctors stop engaging with their patients? Would it matter that much or would we be praised for reaching financial targets and improving throughput? The constant frustration for many nurses is the lack of time they have to be with their patients. Until such functions as support, reassurance, comfort and caring can be quantified it seems that policy makers and managers do not value and therefore do not fund them. Do we have to prove their value from a clinical, scientific base or can we declare them as basic rights for every patient, and as such ought they to be the foundation stones of professional education and evaluations of the quality of patient care?'*

In an RHC project discussion group caring was seen as undervalued. This was not just an issue for the NHS: the care of children or elderly people were also felt to be under-valued occupations. It was also recognized that care was not always valued by patients – or at least the caring and curing could be separated, with expectations of the NHS focused on the latter. The anonymous efficiency or accessibility of the walk in centre or the quick fix of day surgery have their attractions.

The concern was for those who needed care and did not get it or were short-changed with the 'pseudo-relationships' of customer care, devoid of real encounter or commit-ment. An old British Rail description of passengers as 'self-loading freight' was felt to capture the patient throughput culture. The constraints on the relationship with patients was seen as one of the main inhibitors to care, as well as a perceived diminution in the culture of care within medical professions.

In a parallel project to RHC, on residential and nursing care for elderly people, the framework of relational proximity (see Table 4.1) was found to be helpful in identi-fying a set of preconditions which could foster the development of caring relationships and provide a means of assessing how structures and working practices were affecting the care environment. Table 6.1 sets out some of the issues addressed. While they were developed with a particular focus on the residential care of elderly people, many apply to healthcare relationships.

Caring is partly a matter of values and commitment, but it is all too easily under-mined. There is scope for much more work on assessing the quality of caring relation-ships and their medical benefits, and monitoring the impact of working practices, organizational structures, the physical environment and skills and training on the development of caring relationships.

Relational delivery

Relational health requires relational delivery. Without it, integrated care of the whole person cannot happen. Any one patient's experience may involve a complex web of direct and supporting relationships, governed by different models and expectations, facing different constraints, with different objectives and of varying quality. The front-line of therapeutic relationships may comprise many relationships including, for example, several doctors of varying seniority and specialism and working for different organizations, different nurses (and different kinds of nurse) and various professions allied to medicine. But healthcare, in its broadest sense, is not the sole preserve of the medical professions. To the list of healthcare participants may be added home helps, family carers, alternative practitioners, etc.

Behind the frontlines of care provision lie the network of supporting relationships between individuals, teams, professions and organizations. In theory, particularly in the new NHS, they should ensure that the multiplicity of frontline relationships add up to integrated, seamless care for the whole person. The implementation is rarely so simple. The RHC project's discussion group on collaborative relationships was in many ways a rather depressing experience as it recognized that decades of research and discussion had achieved only modest progress in practice. There was not much opti-mism for the future.

Table 6.1. Sample checklist of aspects of care relationship [Source: Relationships Foundation (1998): *Residential Care Home Relational Pack*, unpublished draft training materials]

Directness
► Responsiveness to requests for help
► Access to people for information/advice
► Hearing information first hand
► Open and honest communication
► Opportunities for conversation which go beyond the superficial

Continuity
► Time spent with residents (and factors influencing this)
► Handovers between staff to maintain continuity of care
► Continuity of care with other providers
► Use of key workers or named nurses
► Staff turnover or use of short-term agency staff

Multiplexity
► Awareness of medical, social, emotional and spiritual needs of residents
► Understanding of domestic/family circumstances
► Resident's understanding of staff roles and constraints on what they can do
► Information exchange between staff to build broader understanding of residents
► Opportunities to discover resident's skills, capacities, interests

Parity
► Extent of choice about all aspects of resident's life, eg meal times and bedtimes
► Extent of dignity, courtesy and respect
► Existence and use of complaints procedures
► Participation in care plans and in the running of the home

Commonality
► Shared goals for care
► Shared values and tolerance of diversity
► Empathy

There is agreement on some of the main obstacles and essential preconditions for effective collaboration. At its weakest collaboration can mean little more than working together in some general way. Where collaboration represents a concerted effort to overcome weaknesses in service provision it tends to involve greater coordination or even integration of services. Distinguishing features of collaborative relationships would include some distinction of identity, role or responsibility alongside a clear common purpose and some surrender of control, finances, staff time or loyalty as part of the common endeavour.

Obstacles to collaboration have been extensively researched and discussed. They are not always static and may vary according to the particular form of collaboration, the context and environment at that time. Frequently cited obstacles (e.g. Meads 1997; Hudson, 1998) include:

► working practices

► organizational structures and cultures

► professional cultures and training

► misunderstanding and poor communication

► territoriality and tribalism – defending power, status and influence

▶ funding systems

▶ low morale and work and financial pressures

▶ geography and the lack of coterminosity

There are different forms of collaboration and there may be different routes to achieving it. Principles that are frequently set out include:

▶ *Building reciprocal understanding.* Misunderstanding of role, culture, team structure, accountability, authority, work pressures and organizational constraints seriously hinder collaboration, as do assumptions of homogeneity within professions and organizations. Seeing the other at work (cross-training), creating time and space for discussion, multiprofessional education, organizational and interorganizational development, and fostering attitudes of generosity (Iles 1996) are some of the suggestions for dealing with this.

▶ *Establishing win–win scenarios.* The presumption of altruism is often regarded as an insufficient basis for widespread effective collaboration. While there is plenty of goodwill and commitment to public service around, collaboration is easier when it is structured so that both parties receive some benefit in exchange for the surrender of control.

▶ *Establishing clear common purpose.* Unclear priorities demotivate collaboration by making the task appear too big and hindering identification of early successes or benefits. Where real goals (as opposed to stated goals) and strategies are not shared, collaborative relationships can become a focus for conflict.

▶ *Building individual, professional and organizational capacity not only to tolerate but also to celebrate diversity.* The scale and pace of change in health policy, technology, service configuration and delivery and organizational arrangements can lead to destructive division within as well as between professions and organizations. Becoming more skilled in working with diversity, a question now exercising businesses whose operations are increasingly global, is important.

▶ *Building esteem and respect.* Defensiveness and low morale hinder collaboration. Collaboration may need to be built on a history of rivalry, conflict and negative stereotyping. Creating the confidence and openness to change and to look to the future and not just the past may require considerable effort at personal, professional and organizational levels.

Healthcare requires effective teamwork, yet as Chapter 7 argues, teamwork in primary care lags behind virtually every other public service sector (see p92). A review of the relationships within a nurse-led primary care in Essex pilot was an important reminder that relationships are more difficult than people may expect. All had, not surprisingly, embarked on the pilot with very positive expectations of the relationships that would develop within the team. Their experience, six months in, was consistently slightly worse than expected. Commonality in the relationship was less than expected: the expectation of identical goals was experienced as 'similar goals'. Service priorities were only 'similar' as opposed to the expectation of 'very similar' priorities. Team identity was less than expected and the diversity of their different professions was not the valued resource that was hoped, but something to be tolerated or accommodated. The understanding of each other's work and skills was only 'adequate' rather than 'good' or 'very good'. Significantly, the expectation of investing time up front to build the relationship had not materialized. Understanding was being gained as they went along but the expectation of meeting to discuss work two or three times a week proved to be only two or three times a month. Some tensions and uncertainty were evident in the relationships which were not as open as initially expected. This is in part a normal reflection of optimistic, or even idealistic, expectations being modified in real life and the recognition that relationships take time and effort to build. But perhaps the most important lesson is that for all the theory, real-life relationships always bring their surprises. Unfortunately, for collaboration the surprise is that it is usually more difficult than expected and that the good intentions of relationship building are all too easily squeezed out by operational pressures.

The cultural change of the new NHS, with its greater expectation of collaboration, and the development of new primary care organizations, which may create a better forum for collaboration, offer some hope for the future. What is not yet clear is where the focus for integration will be. Advocates of patient-centred care may point to the patient. Articulate, empowered patients, or those able to pay for the services they want, may be able to get the service to collaborate around them. Vulnerable patients may be focused on, but it seems unrealistic to expect them to focus a health service that cannot integrate itself. Nor will it be easy for health professionals to provide a single focus. The points of entry into the system are now too diverse (GPs are no longer the sole gatekeepers) and no one profession has the necessary breadth of experience of overview. Yet if we accept the reality that integrated care will involve a number of points of focus or convergence, then the health service will need far greater relational maturity than it currently displays. Systems can help or hinder the process, yet are unlikely to provide an adequate solution. RHC will need development, yet, as Chapter 7 argues, the NHS's internal capacity for development has been significantly diminished.

Summary

The relational dimension of health is too often neglected. The links between relationships, stress, social support and disease indicate that the relational fabric of society will be an important factor in the success of addressing public priorities such as CHD or mental health. It also means that caring, too often constrained by the nature of the relationships that are developed with patients, needs to be valued again and fostered. Delivering relational health requires effective relationships between those involved in delivery. Collaboration remains patchy and there are many obstacles to achieving it. Progress will require investment in development.

References

Baker N, ed (1996). *Building a Relational Society*. Aldershot: Arena.

Berkman L *et al* (1992). Emotional support and survival after myocardial infarction: a prospective population based study of the elderly. *Annals of Internal Medicine*. **117**: 12 pp 1003–1010

Boorse C (1981). On the distinction between disease and health. In: Caplan A *et al*, eds. *Concepts of Health and Disease*. Addison Wesley: 554–560.

Bradshaw A (1994). *Lighting the Lamp; The Spiritual Dimension of Nursing Care*. London: Scutari Press.

Bruggen P (1997). *Who Cares? True Stories of the NHS Reforms*. Charlbury: Jon Carpenter Publishing.

Caplan R *et al* (1975) *Job Demands and Worker Health* cited in Argyle M (1996) 'The effects of relationships on well-being' in Baker N (ed) Building a Relational Society Aldershot: Arena pp 33–47.

Department of Health (1998). *National Service Framework for Coronary Heart Disease*, HSC 1998/218. London: Department of Health.

Engel G (1981). The need for a new medical model: a challenge for biomedicine. In: Caplan A *et al*, eds. *Concepts of Health and Disease*. Addison Wesley

Farrell C and Gilbert H (1996). *Health Care Partnerships*. London: King's Fund Publishing.

Fulford K *et al* (1996). *Essential Practice in Patient-Centred Care*. Oxford: Blackwell Science.

Goleman D (1995). *Emotional Intelligence*. London: Bloomsbury: Ch 11.

Guttmacher S (1979). Whole in body, mind and spirit; holistic health and the limits of medicine. In: *Hastings Centre Report*, The Hastings Centre vol. 9: 15–20.

Hudson R (1998). *Primary Care and Social Care*. Leeds: Nuffield Institute.

Iles V (1996). *Really Managing Health Care*. Buckingham: Open University Press.

Ironson G (1992). Effects of anger on left ventricular ejection fraction in coronary artery disease. *American Journal of Cardiology* **70**: 3 pp 281–286

Jubilee Centre (1988). *Biblical Perspectives on Health and Health Care Relationships*. Cambridge: Jubilee Centre.

Kennedy S, Kiecolt-Glaser J and Glaser R (1988) 'Immunological consequences of acute and chronic stressors; mediating role of interpersonal relationships'. *British Journal of Medical Psychology* 62 pp 77–85

Kitson A (1996). A nurse's perspective. In: Fulford K *et al*, eds. *Essential Practice in Patient-Centred Care*. Oxford: Blackwell Science. pp x–xi

Klein R (1995). *The New Politics of the NHS*. London: Longman: 230.

Laura R and Heaney S (1990). *Philosophical Foundation of Health Education*. London: Routledge.

Lynch J (1977). *The Broken Heart*. Basic Books.

Macklin R (1973). The medical model in psychoanalysis and psychotherapy. *Comprehensive Psychiatry* **149**: 172–90

Meads G, ed (1997). *Health and Social Services in Primary Care*. London: Financial Times Healthcare.

McEwen B and Stellar E (1993). Stress and the individual: mechanisms leading to disease. *Archives of Internal Medicine* **153**:

Mittleman M (1994). Triggering of myocardial infarction onset by episodes of anger. *Circulation* **89**(2): p 936

Rosengren A *et al* (1993). Stressful life events, social support, and mortality in men born in 1993. *British Medical Journal* **307** No 6912, pp 1102–1106

Secretary of State for Health (1997). *The New NHS: Modern, Dependable*. London: HMSO.

Sharkey P (1992). *A Philosophical Examination of the History and Values of Western Medicine*. Edwin Mellen Press.

Thoreson C (1990). Anxiety in women and heart disease. In: *Proceedings of the International Congress of Behavioural Medicine*, Uppsala. Cited in Goleman D (1995).

7
Development

*'So I saw that there is nothing better for a man than to enjoy
his work, because that is his lot.
For who can bring him to see what will happen
after him?'*

(Ecclesiastes 3: 22)

Context

Let us now go back just over a decade, before the revolution of the NHS internal
market changes in 1989/1990, and turn to any copy of the *Health Service Journal* at
random. Volume 98 number 5088 published on 18 February 1988 is our *ad hoc* selection. It seems a long time ago. Tony Newton was the Health Minister. A central feature
of this edition is devoted to Leon Brittan's radical proposals for revamping the NHS
through a private sector-led national health insurance scheme. The journal's editorial
line is deeply sceptical. The remaining articles concentrate on secondary care and
financial issues almost exclusively.

Dispersing development

Turn to the back pages for the advertisements. There are 110 for vacant posts. Only two
of these are in what would then have been understood as primary care: a practice
manager's post in Chelmsford and a research role with the Department of General
Practice at St Mary's Hospital Medical School in London. Interestingly, Liverpool
City Council was looking to recruit its own Health Cities project coordinator, courtesy
of combined WHO/European Commission funding: a sign of the times to come. There
are seven posts advertised with 'development' or 'education' in their job titles,
denoting a direct responsibility for enhancing staff performance, and no fewer than 10
'personnel officer' or 'personnel manager' advertisements – 15% of the total. The NHS
in 1988 was self-evidently organized to look after its own. Development was its direct
responsibility.

This edition of the *Health Service Journal* carried no tender documents and only one
advertisement for an external course. This was scheduled to last no less than 13 weeks
on the use of 'Information in the Planning and Evaluation of Health Care Services'. Its
principal targets in terms of recruitment were listed as 'senior NHS medical, nursing
and administrative staff'.

Let us now go forward 10 years and at random pick up the 1998 *Health Service
Journal* volume 108 number 5632, published on 26 November 1998. The first feature
asks whether or not political devolution will signify the end of a 'truly' national health

service and the other three are headed 'primary care', 'public health' and 'integrated care'– clearly a very different subject focus from that of the previous decade.

There are 65 posts advertised this time. The advertisements are noticeably larger and glossier. Nine are for posts in primary care. Only two refer to 'personnel' in the job title but there are five invitations to tender, 25 advertisements for external consultancies and inserts for 19 learning events of which all except three take the form of one-day conferences and events. Of the 19, only two were offered by NHS organizations, the rest being hosted by the independent sector, which also figures as the prospective employer in five of the job advertisements. In total there are 22 non-NHS agencies explicitly offering staff and service development services to the NHS.

Development roles and responsibilities have been transformed within the space of a decade. The outcome of the 1997 general election has made no discernible difference. The trend remains the same. The current issue of the *Health Service Journal* (22 May 1999) contains 32 advertisements in primary care and 23 for external consultancy-style services. The transfer of resource management functions to primary care seems inextricably linked to the dispersal of NHS development capabilities. The two have progressed in tandem and the correlation, at least, is undeniable. What is less certain is the impact. Has the changing profile of development activity signified a new value-for-money variety of support services, engaging, for example, the new universities and pharmaceutical companies in a novel and creative way which is to their mutual benefit? Or does it signal an abrogation of duty? Does the language of 'deploying (or more usually redeploying) human resources' rather than 'developing personnel' mean that the NHS is no longer approaching its overall development, from a relational perspective, in an integrated way that promotes both the health of its staff and those they serve?

Role of the health professions

What is apparent from an analysis of contemporary health policy is that development has become defined by it objects: management, organizations and, most frequently, the professions. The latter have enjoyed something of a comeback in the post-1997 new NHS, although on rather different terms from those enjoyed a decade ago. They are now charged with the responsibility for ensuring central policies are delivered. Management and leadership are no longer terms associated with the exclusively executive roles. As the central guidance on *Developing the Workforce* states:

> 'Managing radical change needs effective leadership. It requires the involvement and commitment of organisations, authorities and staff at all levels and across all agencies'.

> (Department of Health 1999a)

For the professions, as the circular's covering letter emphasizes, there is no hiding place.

> 'The objectives [of Modernising Health and Social Services] in relation to health professions . . . require direct action by Education Consortia and the individual organisations that constitute them'.

Returning NHS development responsibilities to the clinical professionals and care practitioners, accordingly, is not quite what might have been expected; not least by those individuals themselves. It is a tough deal, creating a new implicit contract between the politician and professional. The underlying message is: 'how you develop services to achieve set objectives is down to you; but the objectives are set and we at the centre are setting them'.

The relational perspective

Divorcing development

In this context monitoring remains the big brother to development, just as much as it did when both were functions of dedicated NHS performance management roles in regional and district health authorities between 1992 and 1996. This was a time when lip service only was paid to the even balance between development and monitoring. Of course, the two should be interdependent: the results of monitoring service activity trends, variations in health status and, above all, downturns in financial performance, should help identify not just the priorities but the processes requiring development; and trigger the appropriate enabling support. In reality this cycle of facilitation existed in theory only for most parts of the NHS. Monitoring was 95% of performance management in practice. Performance shortfalls spawned issues of survival rather than support. The sense of development as a noun in its own right, defined without reference to its objects, was almost completely lost. Development ceased to be a legitimate NHS subject and, as the analysis above of *Health Service Journal* advertisements suggests, it was usually a function transferred out of the organization.

Reintegrating development

A relational perspective restores this legitimacy. It recognizes that it is through relationships that the real motivation to make a difference – the essential germ of development – is engendered. Restoring development responsibilities to health professionals and emphasizing their joint agenda with those working in social care goes some way towards acknowledging this perspective. But of itself it does not go far enough; particularly if located within what many in healthcare are now experiencing as a novel and oppressive framework of central regulation and external scrutiny. Enduring developments come from within. They last because they are genuinely owned by their participants. Individuals' values and views come together in a public service through conviction not control. A background of fear – for job security in particular – and coinciding self-interests are not enough. In the public services of healthcare, in particular, with all its personal traumas, professional uncertainties and political overtones, development is a difficult and complex process. It requires sensitivity and patience, time and permission to try and fail and, above all, an absolute, overriding commitment to the relationships with those who are frail and infirm; disabled and dying, diseased, depressed and not infrequently desperate. The nature of these frontline relationships, most numerous and pervasive in primary care settings, should not simply concentrate minds but serve as a focus for developmental activities. More profoundly, they can exist in a condition of symbiosis with the relationships of the health system as a whole; each reinforcing the other.

Development of this kind is precious and rare. Nevertheless, we have found it in some parts of the NHS. In Dorset and the Dunfermline Local Health Care Cooperative, for example, Relational Health Care (RHC) workshops witnessed an unerring identification with the local public so that when healthcare professionals, including NHS managers, looked to their own development requirements it seemed as if these were a direct proxy for the needs of their patients. In such local cultures as these, development is seen as never ending and not a set of time-limited projects. It is an integral part of day-to-day NHS life.

To achieve such a state means a level of development capacity that few NHS organizations have been willing or able to afford and sustain, particularly in the 1998/99 world of 'best value' outsourcing illustrated by the profile of *Health Service Journal* advertisements described above (p83). Development is hard work. It requires time, skills and above all the right attitudes translated into behaviour.

Relational baseline

Table 7.1 is a splendid local example of all these attributes coming together for a primary care group (PCG) development approach – initially in the Southampton and South West Hampshire District in June 1998, but subsequently in Fife, Wolverhampton and a number of other districts. Each used a relational profiling technique in their approach to PCG development. They recognized the relationships challenge inherent in the latter and that this challenge is both long term and on several levels. Self-evidently the relationship between GPs and their practices changes. Indeed, the basic unit of primary care will no longer be 'theirs': in terms of ownership a range of professionals have a legitimate stake in PCGs or trusts.

This implies a significant shift of power, as does the changing relationship with other healthcare providers, particularly the consultants in secondary care settings, with the delegation of contracting and commissioning roles to the new primary care organizations. Also, there are the still only little understood changes in such external relationships as those with local authorities, charities and housing associations. Many of these are also taking on contracting and commissioning responsibilities for the first time; but with significantly different frameworks of accountability and cultures. Finally, there are the potentially radical changes in the relationships with patients and the public. In their case a role reversal may even become possible if, as some predict (Starey 1996, Winkler 1996), future primary care organizations are both membership and franchise based.

Development through participation and encounter

In such an uncertain environment the matrix in Table 7.1 offers a way of working together better to understand and address the alternative scenarios arising from these relationship challenges. It is a classic illustration of development from a relational perspective being put into practice. As such it could scarcely be further away from the clinical, economic and political imperatives detailed in the New NHS white paper

Table 7.1. Developing relationships with PCGs

It is 2001/2002. PCGs are established in each of the health district's (500 000 population) seven local areas, ranging in status from Level 2 to 5, with one having moved beyond Level 4 to incorporate the area social services team. Here discussions on possible local mergers within an enlarged PCT are underway. A specialist joint NHS/Social Services Directorate Mental Health and Special Needs Trust has also been launched. An overall Bureau for Health and Quality meets quarterly and links directly to its central counterparts. It has recently asked the NICE inspectors to visit one local area where the PCG is at Level 2 and there are concerns relating to overall clinical and financial performance. Although the annual resource allocation continues to increase at 2% per annum, in real terms the university hospital's income from PCGs is projected to continue to diminish for three years at an annual rate of 5%. The Labour administration is planning to host one of its regional health assemblies to review progress on its Healthier Nation targets locally if it wins the general election. It is pledged to convert PCGs into genuine 'community organizations' as part of its policy of 'participatory democracy'. Waiting lists continue at around 12 months maximum and reductions in this level are a prerequisite for the granting of 'franchises' by the health authority.

Please identify your PCG's position and status and list your area's six most significant current relationships below, scoring their relative strengths and weaknesses for each relational factor on a 1–5 scale (5 = highest). The factors are as follows:

Commonality:	Shared values and principles
	Complementary aims and objectives
Parity:	Reciprocal respect and worth
	Equity of benefits
Breadth:	Mutual awareness of others' circumstances
	Wide ranging in terms of content, roles and responsibilities
Continuity:	Enduring over time
	Regular interaction
Directness:	Open communications
	Face-to-face contact

Name of organization	Commonality	Parity	Breadth	Continuity	Directness
1.					
2.					
3.					
4.					
5.					
6.					

(Secretary of State for Health 1997). Perhaps revealingly, the chapter in this document which embraces these imperatives as a laudably 'integrated' development agenda requiring the 'duty of partnership' is headed bluntly 'driving change'.

But people do not much like to be driven, unless it is for pleasure, and even then only occasionally. They like to drive themselves and to decide when to do so and where to go. Devising the introductory text of Table 7.1 provided an opportunity for a wide range of new NHS contributors to set the direction. In the Southampton and South West Hampshire exercise, nominated representatives from the health authority, university hospital, general practice, a pharmaceutical company, the NHS community trust and community health council each provided two of the original sentences from which the 2001/2002 scenario was eventually synthesized and agreed. In all 120 participants completed the matrix exercise together, each one taking the opportunity to put themselves in the position of their local PCG to track the changes in its future relationships; and then to revert to type by analysing their host organization's relationship with the emerging PCGs.

Such events develop shared perceptions and judgements. They identify possible ways of addressing shortfalls through, for example, staff exchanges or 'shadowing exercises' to gain a better mutual understanding of each others' roles and responsibilities, or through proposals to pool reserves to share financial risk and demonstrate commitment to a common purpose. In Southampton and South West Hampshire, for example, 'directness' scored very high, but 'commonality' was surprisingly low, especially for a number of organizations with the health authority. They did not see themselves as having shared objectives.

As this dichotomy was explored it became clear that health authority staff could hardly have worked harder to maintain contact and channels of communication. Meetings and memos abounded. The problem was with the style and the source. The health authority, with its three powerful directorates, was in effect externally perceived as three separate and sometimes competing entities, each with its own agendas, terminologies and expectations. As a result of these internal differences 'parity' was hard to achieve and without it the trust and real exchange required for 'commonality' could not be engendered. For PCGs this novel appreciation of the relationships in the overall local health system led to a deeper awareness of how difficult it would be for the health authority to 'let go' and to devolve powers and responsibilities to primary care when issues of parity and commonality were such significant relationship challenges within the authority itself.

A problem of parity

Elsewhere, different profiles emerge in response to different participants' perceptions and different local circumstances. Parity in the NHS is usually low, reflecting differential professional status and when, for example, a version of Table 7.1 was used by the Teeside GP Forum, the continuing cultural expectations of the usually male GP as local king-pin was transferred direct from the surgery to the relational profile of the new PCGs. There are, of course, exceptions. In Camden and Islington 'parity' scores much higher. There is a genuine sense of equivalence if not equality, seemingly engendered by the common feelings of 'being together in the same boat' in terms of all working in a relatively deprived inner-city patch.

In Camden and Islington, however, for the 18 'lead' primary care practitioners drawn from 11 different professions taking part in the local relational profiling exercise, 'breadth' was a real problem. The maximum number of others known to one representative in the group was three. It was clear that while the conditions of Camden served as a leveller, they were also a cause of isolation. The course members recognized this and arranged an afternoon session dedicated to sharing their individual professional backgrounds and future service aims in the context of what each could contribute to the forthcoming PCGs.

Dealing with discontinuity

In Camden and Islington the relational profiling exercise was part of a seven-session PCG development programme sponsored by the health authority over nine months. During this period the four health authority staff members who arranged the programme all changed jobs. This experience is not exceptional. In another central London health authority, a relational audit found that the average life expectancy of an organizational role was 18 months and that of its role holder was less than half this.

In West Surrey, the health authority chief executive was sensitive to the negative impact on relationships of the still very recent legacy of a district health authority merger: reconfiguration of NHS trusts, closure of long-stay hospitals and the abolition of a locally thriving GP fundholding scheme with leading-edge total purchasing pilots at its heart. Each of these changes had aroused strong and at time bitter opposition. There had not simply been separate professional camps but several camps within the professions. As a result, the RHC material was used intensively in six sessions over six weeks (Jan–March 1999) separately by the different professional groupings on PCGs, prior to moving into full PCG membership and operation together. This was a wise move in an area where, as in many other places, the 'continuity' element in healthcare relationships had been so severely undermined that remedial action to repair these relationships within the local health system was vital.

We have witnessed similar health authority initiatives in such diverse districts as West Pennine, Fife, Enfield and Haringey, and Kensington, Chelsea and Westminster. Unfortunately, not all health authorities are mature or secure enough to recognize that developing relationships is an essential part of their new strategic regulation roles. Performance monitoring still comes easier and given the conditioning of recent years, much more naturally.

Developing relationships

Table 7.1 represents a relatively sophisticated relational exercise. For a start it involves many different people, many different organizations and many different and sometimes conflicting perceptions contributing to the relational analysis. If relationships are to be our starting point in identifying the source for development we need to go back a few steps and start with the individual and the individual relationships. Motivation, especially in the public services, needs to be seen as a personal property; not a "calculative commitment" and certainly not as mere compliance. The latter is often the antithesis to health. When compliance is the norm then the resultant relationships automatically inhibit those charged with delivering better health and healthcare.

Starting with individuals

Recognizing the individual as the starting point has been an important part of the RHC approach to PCG development. Traditionally, general practices have been small, singular and separate. They have kept to themselves and not had much to do with the rest of those in the NHS. The move to PCGs has, therefore, come as a giant 'leap in the dark' for most healthcare staff. Feelings of anxiety, suspicion and even hostility have been inevitable. Central policy statements have scarcely mentioned this dimension of personal dilemmas. Asserting the self-evident correctness of policy has been enough to legitimize, in some cases, major new powers with few of the conventional NHS checks and balances. For example, the central guidance on *Developing Primary Care Groups* is turned in its preamble into a highly specific and detailed 'agenda for action' (Department of Health 1998). In terms of their core responsibilities for community services development, public health improvement and hospital services commissioning the statement is bald:

> *'Primary Care Groups must be vehicles for decision making not just maintaining the status quo **whatever the need for change'**.*

The emphasis is ours. In the original text the whole sentence is in bold type as is the 'agenda for action'. The sense of an instruction requiring obedience, if not compliance, seems unmistakable. The previous government's circulars, by contrast, were littered with the words 'choice' and 'diversity'. They rarely appear now.

Preparing for primary care

Given this sense of righteousness about what PCGs are for, what further persuasion for their development could be needed? Of course, in reality, the answer is that the real development needs remain substantial, as illustrated by Table 7.2. It sets out a simple checklist of the areas of knowledge and experience that are valuable for individuals to possess if they are to take forward a health system in which the principal focus is becoming primary care. It is not an exhaustive list, but is sufficient to be credible and as such has been used by more than 20 NHS organizations and training courses: enough to start to see an overall pattern emerging in the local responses.

It is possible for individuals completing the checklist to score a total of 100. Only twice, in fact, have we seen 70 exceeded. We have witnessed some disarmingly low scores, some of which are by respondents of whom more might have been expected and of whom a great deal more will be expected if PCGs and the 'new NHS' are to deliver on its claims. For example, most senior health authority staff score between 20 and 25; the exceptions are mainly those with a family health services authority or family practitioner committee background. Board members of NHS community trusts fare no better, although if they complete the exercise with each other, rather than individually, the score rises to around 40, suggesting a lack of confidence and morale in those organizations for which the NHS as a whole still seems to have little clear purpose. NHS acute trusts score below the 20 points mark but, alarmingly, so do individual NHS training officers and management consultants. This really does highlight the lack of appropriate development capacity within the new NHS.

Across the different groupings there are some signs of common trends. The very lowest scores are reserved for the areas of devolution to patients, family health services contracts and interprofessional education. The tenth item virtually always scores the highest: 'a commitment to primary care-centred policy'. Everybody believes in the focus on primary care, even if most have relatively little idea as to what this means, let alone how they can help achieve it. The only consistent high scorers on the checklist have been members of primary care teams with a background in fundholding; which is

Table 7.2. Preparing for an NHS focused on primary care: self-assessment test

Please give yourself an honest score of between 1 and 10 on each of the following, with higher scores indicating strengths. No nil scores are allowed

Score

i)   Background in community-based services
ii)   Involvement with primary care teams
iii) Understanding of family health services contracts
iv) Contribution to health and social services collaboration
v)   Work with independent sector (ie voluntary, private)
vi) Support for development of primary care-led commissioning
vii) Service shifts from secondary care
viii) Participation in interprofessional education
ix) Devolved responsibilities to patients
x)   Commitment to primary care-centred NHS policy

Total

[Based on Meads (1997)].

now being summarily abolished. The potential gap between intention and implementation is obvious. Currently theirs is the most fragile of relationships.

Fragile relationships, central solutions

The awareness of this fragility tends to produce an increase in centrally prescribed solutions; as those with responsibility for policy strive to ensure its translation into practice. *The New NHS* white paper is unequivocal that the delivery of healthcare is 'a matter of local responsibility':

> *'Local doctors and nurses who are in the best position to know what patients need will be in the driving seat in shaping services.'*
>
> (Secretary of State for Health 1997, p11)

But this is not how the experience of the new NHS has communicated itself to us in our roles as participant observers. More apparent than any sense of local liberation of professionals is, for example, the new requirement from October 1999 on all NHS providers and authorities to:

> *'conduct a baseline self-assessment of compliance with risk management and organisational controls standards'*

in which formal signed assurances in respect of clinical governance are the first requirement' (Department of Health 1999b). We are told the development task for every NHS organisation is 'a comprehensive control framework', the precise structure and operational format of which will be centrally defined. There may appear to be a bizarre mismatch between, for example, a single novice National Institute for Clinical Excellence (NICE) reliant on the limited evidence and constrained methodologies of clinical trials, cohort studies and systematic reviews on the one hand, and the accumulated experience of general practice's 750 000 individual consultations each day on the other. Despite this, however, the desire to make things happen through central initiatives continues apace.

But development cannot be forced. It is neither compulsory nor compulsive. When vertical relationships supersede those between peers, particularly when converted into contractual forms, the development process is undone. The trust needed for productive lateral relationships is both threatened and inhibited through the lack of confidence and faith shown in them by the burden and content of top-down communications. If this persists for a period the vertical relationships will themselves scarcely exist as relationships at all; except on paper. All this provides a deeply unsatisfactory model of developing relationships within the health system to apply to the relationships of healthcare between those local nurses and doctors cited in *The New NHS* quotation above and their patients.

Getting started

It is almost as if the new NHS needs to be deconditioned. The experience of the RHC project over the 1996–99 period at local levels has often been that of going back to the beginning. Table 7.3 is an example of a simple exercise drawing on the relationships profiling approach described in Chapter 4, used by NHS trust board members and fundholding GP 'leads' in parts of central London and Suffolk in 1997. This helped them come to terms with the new NHS by looking into the mirror and seeing who they had become as a result of the internal market period in relation to their neighbours. Sometimes the insularity of a NHS unit is truly staggering. For example, on university courses it is still possible today to teach relatively senior clinicians and managers who remain unaware that fundholding is being abolished (or even what it was); and who are completely unaware of developments beyond their local district, let alone within a UK-wide or international context. In this environment Table 7.3 at least provides a basis for dialogue and learning together. It is also a useful benchmarking exercise by which future progress can be measured. As such it is valuable to employ it in sequence with Tables 7.1 and 7.4 or 7.5.

Tables 7.4 and 7.5 represent the next steps in getting started. Both again are live examples and provide simple frameworks for local relationship-based development. Each enabled those involved in local primary care leadership roles to move on from individual self-definition in relation to others to collective self-development in conjunction with others. Again both approaches are very straightforward, so at this stage it is important to remind ourselves that in terms of such relational practices as teamwork, primary care has constantly lagged behind virtually every other public service sector (Ovretveit and Elwyn 1998).

A classic contemporary study, for example, which used joint development and shared objectives as two if its key criteria, found the GP-based primary health care team in last place behind its counterparts in social work, community mental health and nursing (Poulton and West 1993). Other than in rebellions against such central policy or legislative initiatives as the new national contracts of 1990 (Klein 1995, pp200–1), family health services professionals do not have a significant history of working together. In relational terms the new NHS is placing the 'duty of partnership' (Secretary of State for Health 1997, p45) with those who have perversely used the term most in the past, but who often have the least experience of what it means, ie GPs.

Table 7.3. Facing up to the future

It is the 1997/98 NHS annual cycle. The pre-May 1997 arrangements continue to apply (eg annual contracts, fundholding, etc). Please list your organization/sector's six most significant current relationships below and score their relative strengths and weaknesses for each relational factor on a 1–5 scale (5 = highest). The factors are as follows:

Commonality: Shared values and principles
                 Complementary aims and objectives
Parity: Reciprocal respect and worth
                 Equity of benefits
Breadth: Mutual awareness of others' circumstances
                 Wide ranging in terms of content, roles and responsibilities
Continuity: Enduring over time
                 Regular interaction
Directness: Open communications
                 Face-to-face contact

Name of organization	Commonality	Parity	Breadth	Continuity	Directness
1.					
2.					
3.					
4.					
5.					
6.					

Share your assessments with colleagues from your own and other organizations. Identify and discuss common perceptions and differences and, if possible, suggest steps that may be taken to develop The *New NHS* together.

This last statement rings particularly true in Cambridgeshire, with its deeply conservative primary care culture, where a modified version of Table 7.4 was introduced at an early meeting of PCGs and health authority staff and members toward the end of 1998. This is a county where there has been continuous change at health authority level and at different times over the past 10 years the number of authorities has ranged from one to five. The turnover at this level has contrasted with relative stability in primary care personnel. Practices have been able to defend themselves against continuous change by being self-reliant. Fundholding levels were always low, with very few consortia-type initiatives. It is a good place now both to start with the grassroots on the one hand and to be hard headed about the need to sustain performance before extending it on the other. It is also a good place to start in terms of the need to revive relationships across the county's healthcare system.

The results of completing a Table 7.4-type exercise invariably convert the principle of subsidiarity from a defence mechanism into a source of potential interdependence. Not that much is entered in the 'practice' box in the matrix and at PCG/health authority

Table 7.4. Getting started: A workshop exercise for PCG board members, with local health authority support

The purpose of this exercise is to help PCG members address their new strategic functions, understanding strategy as requiring both clarity of direction in terms of the key tasks to be undertaken and effective relational processes. The exercise helps each PCG define itself as a distinctive primary care organization through its working partnerships.

The exercise is as follows:

a) List your (previously agreed) local strategic priorities for development
b) Then complete the following matrix at your designated PCG level (eg Level 2), drawing on your previously identified local priorities, and central guidance. The latter confirms PCG main areas of responsibility as being:

▶ improvements in community health
▶ developments in primary and community care
▶ commissioning of secondary and associated services
▶ PCG organizational development

PCG level(s)	Practice	Inter-practice	Intra-PCG	Inter-PCG	PCG/HA
eg 2 (ie health authority subcommittee)	eg prescribing protocols	eg clinical governance			
eg 4 (i.e. NHS primary trust)				eg quality programmes	eg managed care regimes

c) Then list and classify the priorities above in the following categories:

A = Must do   (1998/1999)
B = Will do   (1999/2000)
C = Would like to do   (2000/2001)
D = Will not do   (2001/2002)

d) Repeat exercise at another selected PCG level (eg Level 3) and discuss differences in terms of impact on local aims and relationships

level the items are also of an exceptional character, warranting significant but intermittent contact. It is the middle sections of the matrix that get filled up, moving progressively towards the right-hand side as the PCG level rises from 1 to 4. At Level 4 the PCG or trust is *the* local health organization and its relationships with its direct counterparts, therefore, are crucial in the full range of decisions, from what must to what will not be done.

In Wales, as yet, there are no different formal levels of PCGs and the emerging primary care organizations are differently constituted. These local health groups (LHG), for example, must be based on the boundaries of local authorities, which are strongly represented in the LHG membership of 18 as compared with between 10 and

13 in England (Secretary of State for Wales 1998). Community pharmacists in Wales are core members; in England they are not. In Wales there is no provision for direct commissioning responsibilities; in England this, in financial terms at least, will be the first role of a NHS primary care trust (PCT). In the Welsh context, accordingly, the climate is more conducive at this stage to using the advent of LHGs as a classic 'learning organization' opportunity (Senge 1990), exploring tomorrow's futures by synthesizing today's experiences. There are not quite the same operational pressures and demands as over the border. LHGs can explore and develop together – on the level, as it were.

Table 7.5 is an illustration of this approach, and again provides a very simple way in to a relational perspective on development. It was being applied by individual LHGs in South and West Wales in 1998. The local participants were taken aback by the results. As fiercely patriotic and proud of their surgeries and health centres as any other native group, the GPs in, for example, the Wrexham area found that virtually no major development priorities remained at the individual practice level. Of the nine identified objectives in Table 7.5, moreover, it is usually hard to identify more than one or two (eg staff development, managing the finances) where the principal focus of action does not move to the relationship between pairs of LHGs, if not beyond. The new NHS in Wales promises to be a profoundly educative experience.

Educational endings

The relational approach to development is, of course, more about education than training. New skills and techniques – such as those set out in the Tables above – may help but they represent the tactics not the strategy. The latter targets the attitudes that fundamentally affect behaviour and the views and values these comprise. These are the educational end points for relationships based development. The assertion that the NHS has been developed largely and traditionally through its distinctive and separate professions has often been made both in theory and in practice (Klein 1995, pp49–52, 86–7, Webster 1998). Moreover, in the UK, unlike in much of the rest of Europe, the liberal professions convey a social (and financial) status and autonomy of lifestyle that it would be almost unnatural for individuals not to want to preserve and protect. This is

Table 7.5. Making local health groups (LHGs) work: Draft local health group objectives for 1999/2000. List your LHG's objectives. Indicate whether the principal focus of action lies with individual LHGs or with LHGs together.

Objectives	Each LHG	LHGs together
Establish an effective LHG		
Manage the finances		
Further develop joint working		
Establish effective waiting list management		
Further develop primary care		
Develop input to long-term agreements		
Develop input to health improvement programme		
Establish clinical governance arrangements		
Staff development		

one reason why general managers have frequently felt the need to be either autocratic or powerfully political when faced with the need to deliver overall corporate objectives expeditiously. It also helps explain why, as illustrated on p89, a background in inter-professional education scores so poorly with so many as a prerequisite for progressing a new NHS focused on primary care. We are not used to the relationships of learning together except with those of our own kind.

Interprofessional education

This is a problem about which something is now being done. It is possible to point to some new universities where the majority of postgraduate programme curricula have interprofessional spines (eg Oxford Brookes), where information technology is being used with great imagination to draw different professionals into shared learning experiences (eg Derby) and where there are hub-and-spoke partnerships with networks of local colleges and NHS units to promote integrated-care developments (eg Bournemouth). But these are still very much on the margin, the exceptions to the rule of unidisciplinary and uniprofessional courses and qualifications. Many of the longer-standing academic institutions have hardly changed at all, and lacking their support the national Centre for the Advancement of Inter-Professional Education (CAIPE) stumbles from one financial crisis to another. Symbolically, somehow, this seems to speak volumes. In 1999 CAIPE's central NHS funding was withdrawn just as the multipro-fessional PCGs began to emerge.

Unfortunately and predictably, the educational response of the new NHS has been largely structural. There are the new national service frameworks to tell you what to do in terms of clinical and cost-effectiveness on the one hand (Secretary of State for Health, p57) and the organizational consortia of regional education development groups (Secretary of State for Health, p52) to prepare you for action on the other. The latter are in their very early stages, still tied for the most part to long-term provider contracts for nursing and the individual therapies, the national organizations for which remain reluctant to give their accreditation to an individual award-bearing module or programme unless its course content is predominantly, or even exclusively, drawn from their individual disciplines.

City University in London is in this respect like many others. The module titles can be deceptive. 'Health Care Ethics', 'Quality of Life' and 'Philosophy of Healthcare' sound like the right sort of nomenclatures. Nominally, the student intake for these modules is open and generic. In practice, the material presented and approved by the NHS professional bodies is only for nurses, economists and psychologists, respec-tively. The education establishment will not change until it is sure the NHS has. Over the past decade especially the latter has had too many fashions and the result is too little trust and understanding. Once again the relationship issue is at the heart of the problem.

Development requires real education, not 'quick fix' training

Recognizing this in terms of moving the new NHS forward does help with its educa-tion. The latter can and should be about first principles. Relationships and behaviour qualify as such; transient organizations and even more enduring units of professionals

Table 7.6. Interactive types of learning

▶ Exchange based	(eg debates, games)
▶ Action based	(eg problem solving, group exercises)
▶ Observation	(eg site visits, shadowing)
▶ Simulation	(eg role play, action learning sets)
▶ Practice based	(eg placements, assignments)

(Source: Barr H, keynote address: Interactive learning. European Multi-Professsional Education Annual Conference, Maastricht, 1998)

do not. On these foundations as, for example, Barr's (1994) pioneering work has recognized, it is possible to develop. Table 7.6 lists a typology of interactive learning approaches based on his work at Westminster and Greenwich Universities. It is hierarchic with each stage overlapping. Exchanges, educationally designed, encourage a mutual appreciation. They begin to break down barriers not least – in terms of the NHS – arising from distinct and separate professional terminologies to establish one language. Shared experiences provide the material for action learning so that, for example, health visitors and social workers can recognize their own and each other's contributions to child protection or the care of a frail elderly person. They can help reinforce the common ground from which the opportunities for collaboration will grow. Relationships-based development requires the healthcare system to put aside the quick fixes of training consultancies and rediscover the value of real education. Unfortunately, for some universities this statement is equally true and applicable.

It would be Machiavellian to suggest that the New NHS is designed to be disingenuous in its approach to development. Activity may seem to contradict the principles proclaimed to be enabling – decentralization, partnership and integration – but it would be harsh to allege it is deliberately so. The local NHS is still ambivalent. It is sensitive to ambiguities, sometimes when they genuinely exist and sometimes where they do not. The energy, as we approach the millennium with a government keen to make up for lost time, is at the centre. The local NHS is tired. For it development has meant political or economic drivers and above all change, sometimes dressed up as consolidation. Change is inherently ambivalent. It automatically has consequences for relationships, for better or for worse. For worse in healthcare means to the detriment of patient services and public health. These need better relationships. Reassuming responsibilities for these relationships from within the NHS, starting with the individual, progressing through the right sort of relationships and valuing education again, together mean development, as a noun, in its own right.

Summary

The increased concern over NHS relationships has coincided with the decline of development as a NHS role and function. Some PCGs are now assuming responsibility for reversing both trends. Developing robust relationships for health, however, requires sound methodologies. The frameworks of relational proximity and interactive learning are examples of these and offer ways in which the NHS can recover its capacity successfully to develop itself.

References

Barr H (1994). *Perspectives on Shared Learning*. London: Centre for Advancement of Inter-Professional Education.

Department of Health (1998). *The New NHS: Modern and Dependable: Developing Primary Care Groups*, HSC 1998/139. Leeds: NHS Executive: 3–12.

Department of Health (1999a). *Modernising Health and Social Services: Developing the Workforce*, HSC 1999/111, LAC (99)18. Leeds: NHS Executive: 3.

Department of Health (1999b). *Governance in The New NHS*, HSC 1999/123. Leeds: NHS Executive: 2–3.

Klein R (1995). *The New Politics of the NHS*. London: Longman.

Meads G (1997). *Power and Influence in the NHS*. Oxford: Radcliffe Medical Press: 20.

Ovretveit J and Elwyn G (1998). Integrated nursing teams and the PHCT: integral or alternative? In: Elwyn G and Smail J, eds. *Integrated Teams in Primary Care*. Oxford: Radcliffe Medical Press: 37–53.

Poulton P and West M (1997). A failure of function: Teamwork in primary healthcare. *Journal of Interprofessional Care* **11**: 205–16.

Secretary of State for Health (1997). *The New NHS: Modern, Dependable*, Cm3807. London: HMSO.

Secretary of State for Wales (1998). *Putting Patients First*. Cardiff: The Welsh Office: 43–9.

Senge P (1990). *The Fifth Discipline*. London: Century.

Starey M (1996). The primary care trust: Co-ordination for Cohesion. In Meads G, ed. *Future Options for General Practice*. Oxford: Radcliffe Medical Press: 165–90.

Webster C (1998). *The National Health Service. A Political History*. Oxford: Oxford University Press: 12–28.

Winkler F (1996). Collective and individual responsibilities. *Primary Care Management* **6**(7/8): 2–8.

8
Review

'Better what the eye sees than the roving of the appetite.'
(Ecclesiastes 6: 9)

Look while you leap

An NHS in transition must be Janus faced – looking backwards and forwards. If it does not look to the future, if there is no vision, it risks being stuck with the ambiguities and uncertainties of the (present) transition period. The vision may be uncertain and change evolutionary, but progress with no agreed destination – or rather staging post, for no organization's journey ever ends and the horizon may only unfold slowly – is likely to be limited. But looking backwards is also key to going forwards. The course alterations and the learning that enable better progress come from reviewing the past. For a service in transition, and which is likely to remain a more fluid organization than it has been in the past, the review process is of particular importance.

Review is, therefore, a much broader concept than performance management which, in the new NHS, is still struggling to escape the criticisms of too narrow a focus and of creating perverse incentives. Review is, or should be, closely linked to the core functions described in previous chapters.

▶ Policies should be reviewed for their impact and effectiveness. There needs to be a balance between avoiding excessive brakes on innovation while ensuring that policy initiatives do, in fact, achieve desired and desirable outcomes.

▶ Resource allocation and utilization are reviewed to ensure efficiency and fairness.

▶ Strategy requires a regular cycle of review to ensure that it remains inclusive and on track.

▶ Care delivery is reviewed to ensure and improve quality.

As well as supporting individual functions, the process of review links them together by examining the impact of one on the others, and pointing to changes which could make them more mutually supporting.

An inclusive process

Review should also be an inclusive process, involving the whole NHS as well at its external stakeholders such as individual patients, local communities and other agencies including for example, local authorities. External involvement enables participation and provides accountability. The latter is important, but if external monitoring (in this context external may include other NHS organizations) is the only form of review it risks severing the link with learning, development and the consequent improvements in delivery. If review, like quality (see Chapter 9), simply becomes an instrument of control the new NHS will not emerge. Review should therefore include all those involved in service provision, as well as those who are accountable for such issues as clinical effectiveness, public health or financial control.

Review should also involve everyone in the NHS because it should be a personal as well as an organizational discipline. As Iles (1997) has argued, managing yourself as well as managing other people is a responsibility for everyone – not just for people who have the word manager in their job title. Review, in the sense of learning from both success and failure, is as important for personal development as it is for an organization's.

The right tools for the job

The different processes and degrees of participation in review will reflect the range of purposes it serves. This range of purposes is recognized in the new national performance framework issued by the Department of Health (NHS Executive 1998). They are principally associated with informing choice, service improvement (quality, effectiveness and efficiency), strategy [particularly health improvement programmes (HImPs)], commissioning and accountability. This range of purposes, together with the broad focus and participation of review, will require similar breadth in the range of approaches. This is not yet always evident. The concept of review is perhaps most robust and well developed in the areas of clinical research, financial control and performance management. Important as they are, these cultures of review are not necessarily best suited to guiding the new NHS through its transition (Meads 1998). Their strength lies in robust high-level indicators of whether processes are efficient and effective. They are weaker when set in isolation, when they become an end in themselves and when reviewing how the means of strategy, organization and development could better support delivery.

The different purposes of review should use different methodologies and provide different outcomes. The guidance on the local evaluation of personal medical services pilots (NHS Executive 1997), however, produced a hierarchy of the levels of evidence (Table 8.1) drawn directly from the research sector for clinical outcomes and

Table 8.1. Levels of evidence for evaluation of personal medical services pilots

► Randomized controlled trial
► Non-randomized experimental trial
► Non-randomized cohort (observational) study
► Case control (observational) study
► Large differences from comparisons between times and/or places
► Descriptive study

[Source: Meads (1998) adapted from the NHS Centre for Reviews and Dissemination, University of York]

effectiveness. The randomized controlled trial is at the top and the descriptive study is at the bottom.

This does not provide the basis for reviewing how the pilots as organizations and models of delivery have worked or could be improved. Rather this is the terrain of action learning and research (see Chapter 1) which has formed the basis of this project. This chapter, therefore, introduces some of the tools and processes which could be used for reviewing relational health care (RHC), as well as drawing together the conclusions from our review of many parts of the new NHS.

Relational reviews

We have argued that relationships lie at the heart of health and healthcare. They constitute an important aspect of good health, a cause of ill health and an essential element of care provision. This applies both to the frontline relationships between the NHS and patients and the whole range of supporting relationships within and between NHS organizations, as well as with other organizations, eg local authorities. The fact that they are an important focus of current health policies, a key resource – particularly for virtual, stakeholder, community or learning organizations – and an essential element in strategy and care delivery processes, makes them an important focus for review.

Relationships are complicated. That is the starting point of Hinde's (1997) account of the obstacles to a science of interpersonal relationships. In looking at the methodological problems he points out that:

> 'Each dyadic relationship involves two individuals, each with a past history and expectations and hopes for the future; it involves cognitive, affective and behavioural components, each of which influences the other; it exists over time; and it has no clear boundaries, being constantly affected by extra-dyadic influences. It is thus not surprising that the study of relationships is beset by conceptual and methodological difficulties.'

(Hinde 1997, p16)

A science of multilateral relationships between organizations will be no easier and may be expected to encounter the same principal methodological problems listed by Hinde, which include the:

▶ need for subjective data (with all their limitations for hard measures) as well as objective data

▶ difficulty of maintaining a distinction between descriptive and explanatory concepts when 'the characteristics of relationships are explained in terms of processes which are themselves characteristics of the relationship' and where the concepts used have 'woolly edges' as a result of their varied everyday usage

▶ consequences of an analytical approach which may appear to impoverish relationships by describing parts in isolation from the whole and 'intellectualize' the unconscious or partially conscious elements of the relationship

▶ appropriate balance between the complexity of the individual case and the need for generalizations

▶ difficulty of conducting the necessary longitudinal studies

▶ difficulties of controlled-condition experimental approaches in studying real-life relationships

▶ fact that cultural values (including subcultures within a society) will inform what are considered positive and negative relationship traits

▶ multiplicity of generalizations, mini-theories and theories [Hinde (1997), pp16–20].

Work relationships have both personal and organizational dimensions. Where the organisation's relationships are weak, individuals with good personal relationships can make the system work. This is not always and perhaps not usually the case: the consistent failure to achieve more effective collaboration cannot be blamed on the failures of individuals to overcome the problems. Conversely, dysfunctional relationships between individuals can create problems despite a positive relationship between their respective organizations. Developing the personal relationships (and reviewing them as part of this process) is therefore important. The capacity to do this is relatively well established although, as West and Pillinger (1996) have argued in a review of approaches to developing team relationships, not all approaches can be shown to improve performance.

Interpersonal relationships are, however, only half the story and approaches to assessing organizational relationships are much less well developed. Relationships are influenced by their environment – the organizational structures, infrastructures, culture and working practices which can foster or undermine effective relationships. Promoting particular behaviours in an inimical environment is difficult. Policy, resource allocation, strategy, models of care delivery and organizational development will often have far more direct input on this relational environment than on the interpersonal behaviours. Reviewing these functions, therefore, requires a focus on organizational relationships. Frameworks for reviewing relationships may provide useful concepts to help people engage with the complex, and for many people, nebulous concept of relationship and crystallize issues and perceptions. Numerical scores may be generated but, even for the best validated approaches, the review process any tools support is likely to be more important than any quantitative assessment. Relational reviews should not usually be seen as stand-alone processes for a relationship is best reviewed in context – in terms of both its purpose and the external pressures. This is important because the relationship is not (usually) an end in itself. Although relationships are an important and often neglected element of review they cannot replace the review of clinical outcomes or financial performance. Real-life relationships are significantly influenced by external factors and face competing demands and obligations. Hypothetical relationships reviewed out of context do not, in our experience, reveal the tensions which can make relational reviews such a powerful developmental process.

In reviewing relationships there is an extensive range of questions which can be asked (Table 8.2). These have emerged from the many workshops and seminars we have conducted as part of the project. Which are most relevant will depend on the stage of the relationship and the purpose of the review. Different tools and processes may be needed for these different questions. This chapter does not offer a comprehensive toolkit for answering these questions – not least because such toolkits are only recently being developed and can as yet be classified as still work in progress. There is, however, a range of accessible tools and concepts that provide a useful starting point.

Table 8.2. Checklist of questions for reviewing relationships (based on workshop for London Region on tools to support health improvement programmes)

▶ Which relationships are involved?
▶ Which constitute a risk factor (because of their state and importance)?
▶ What would constitute a 'good' relationship in this content? Is this agreed by the parties?
▶ How should the relationship operate? Are these expectations shared?
▶ How is the relationship perceived? Are these perceptions shared? And do they match expectations?
▶ What are the limiting factors (both systems and people)?
▶ Is the relationship producing desired outcomes?
▶ What can be done to develop the relationship?
▶ Is there a commitment to change?
▶ Is the relationship being adequately monitored and managed?

The relational mapping exercise (see Table 7.1) can be used to give an initial indication of which relationships are involved and which are most in need of development. This has proved a useful exercise with health professionals who are coming to terms with the relationship implications of the new NHS. So, for example, we have used it with primary care group (PCG) boards or those involved in developing health improvement programmes (HImPs) to establish a baseline for their current relationships and set a development agenda. Where the mapping exercise is used with a group it can prompt a rich discussion (Table 8.3).

The process of relational mapping is not designed to provide a comprehensive review of the state of any one relationship. It does allow an initial assessment of whether time investment and quality of relationship match relationship priorities; and where the biggest dividends from relationship improvement may be found. To aid the prioritization of relationships this kind of discussion, which typically raises many issues, can be summarized in a matrix (Table 8.4). These issues, and the development needs that emerge from them, require a more focused assessment.

Agreeing the style and structure of the relationship, and reviewing the extent of the agreement about this, is one element of answering the question, What constitutes a 'good' relationship? There is no one answer to this as it will vary according to the context and purpose of the relationship and the participants may legitimately hold different views. There will be a functional element to the answer (a 'good' relationship should be capable of producing desired outcomes, although these may or may not be agreed); an ethical dimension; as well as a personal view ('I like this style of relationship'). The relational proximity framework (Table 8.5) can be used as a basis for negotiating which preconditions are most important.

Table 8.3. Discussion questions arising from relational mapping exercises

1. *Which relationships have been selected*:
▶ Are people agreed? If not, why not?
▶ What are the different reasons for selection? The strategic importance of the relationship? Because delivery will not happen without them? Because of the importance of the client group they represent?
▶ Would the same relationships be selected in five years time? Which become more or less important? How will activities and time allocation change to reflect this? How are relationships of future importance being cultivated?

2. *Which relationships are stronger or weaker?*
▶ Do people agree on scores? If not, does this reflect their different experiences? Or different weighting attached to different aspects of each dimension?
▶ Which of the relationships are notably strong or weak compared to the others? Do they feel the best or the worst? What kind of relationships are they, eg operational or strategic; new or old; interorganizational or interprofessional?
▶ What are the likely consequences of any weakness in these relationships? How can these be mitigated?

3. *Do any dimensions of the relationships tend to be weaker or stronger?*
▶ If so, what are the reasons for this? Does this reflect generic pressures on healthcare relationships (eg cultural or structural issues)?
▶ What are the consequences of weaknesses in these aspects of the relationships? How can they be ameliorated?

Prioritization may reflect the differing importance attached to different outcomes. If, for example, particular importance is attached to improving accountability in a relationship, attention may be focused on such issues as face-to-face communication (it is often easier to dissemble by fax or e-mail), openness and honesty, continuity in the relationship (insufficient communication or high levels of staff turnover may hinder accountability), or issues of power in the relationship. Where new relationships are being established, or they are seen as strategic relationships, RHC project participants have often been most concerned about parity and commonality in establishing the foundations of the relationship. Where the structure of the relationship is a given, and people have been more concerned about its operational effectiveness, the issues of directness, continuity and multiplexity have been more to the fore. This is not to say that in each case the other dimensions are unimportant, but rather that in making the tough choices about where time, energy and attention is going to be focused, some aspects of a relationship will inevitably be accorded more importance than others.

Table 8.4. Matrix for prioritizing relationships

List which relationships are a significant element of your work	How much time per week do you spend on this relationship?	How important is it for your work?	What is the current quality of this relationship?	What impact would improving this relationship have?

Table 8.5. Relational proximity – five preconditions for effective relationships (Source: Relationships Foundation, reproduced with permission)

Precondition	Description
Directness	*Quality of communication process*
Medium	Right medium to maximize amount/quality of information exchange
Access	Direct communication avoiding delay and misunderstandings
Responsiveness	Reliable, quick channels of communication
Style/skills	Communication characterized by listening, openness and honesty
Continuity	*Shared time over time*
Relationship building	Investment of time, developing ways of working effectively
togetherAmount/regularity	Contact in the relationship, keeping abreast of any changes
Length/stability	Consistency in the relationship, continuing commitment to it
Managing change	Maintaining the continuity of the relationship through change
Multiplexity	*Breadth of knowledge*
Organization/department	Work constraints and opportunities for the other, the issues they face
Task/function	Understanding of role and the skills and experience the other brings
Personal understanding	Informal contact; knowledge of personal interests, goals and values
Parity	*Use and abuse of power*
Participation	Involvement in decision making within the relationship
Fair benefits	Arrangements that represent the fair distribution of risk and reward
Fair conduct	Application of standards, treating people with respect and integrity
Commonality	*Valuing similarity and difference*
Shared objectives	Common view of objectives, priorities and means of achieving them
Common culture	Way of working reflects understanding of operating environment
Positive diversity	Recognition of different views, valuing new perspectives
Resolving disagreements	Exploration of difficult issues, finding solutions collectively

Because of the profound nature of the changes taking place in the healthcare environment we have often found that individuals, even as organizational representatives, have drawn on their fundamental experiences of relationships in family life to be able to locate where they are starting from within the new NHS. Accordingly, the concepts and methods of transactional analysis (Bion 1961, Berne 1968) have sometimes proved helpful in their simplicity. Table 8.6 provides an illustration from an earlier NHS project of how the basic interorganizational relationships within the NHS were being perceived by general managers around the time of new Labour's general election victory in 1997. There are also a range of checklists for such different aspects of relationships as partnerships (Devlin 1998), collaboration (Hudson 1998), or participation (Peckham *et al* 1996).

The relational proximity framework (Table 8.5) can also be used to compare expectations and experience of a relationship. Take parity for example. At what point do you expect to be consulted? Are you consulted well in advance, or told about decisions before (or after) they are made, or do you find out about them by chance, eventually? Where do you expect influence or responsibility in a particular relationship to be? Has the distribution of risk and reward been as you expected? Aligning expectations about these in advance can avoid tension and misunderstanding later and can be used to set performance specifications against which a relationship can be reviewed. This

Table 8.6. General managers' perceptions of interorganizational relationships within the NHS

Pre-1990s: familial

| Parent | → | Child, | eg consultants to patients, district health authority to CHC |
| Child | → | Parent, | eg NHS to Department of Health, FHS contractors to HHSA/FPC |

1990s: Immature/transitional

| Child | → | Adult, eg health authorities in deficit with NHS Executive regional offices, new primary care trusts with health authorities |
| Adult | → | Parent, eg trusts with health authorities, NHS Executive with Department of Health |

Post-1990s: mature/prospective

| Adult | → | Adult, eg health authority/general practice fundholder strategic alliances, preferred provider long-term service agreements, regional office market regulation, GP/patient priority setting |

(Meads 1997)
CHC = Community Health Council, FHS = Family Health Services, FHSA = Family Health Services Authority, FPC = Family Practitioner Committee

relatively simple exercise can prompt a whole stream of questions for review and reflection (Table 8.7).

Good review should point to action. Correctly identifying the causal factors that influence the relationship is important in learning from both success and failure. A checklist of factors which all participants can rate for their impact on both their own and their counterpart's contribution to the relationship can help this: an illustrative selection of factors is given in Table 8.8.

If review is to lead to action it helps if some basic principles for making relationships work are accepted and that there is an appropriate process. The principles in Table 8.9 are based around the ideas of Wilmot (1987). Review without an acceptance of the possibility, or even inevitability, of change is less likely to lead to effective action. Relationships should be more dynamic than structures and, as the parties to the relationship change (by virtue of the development of existing parties or the entry of new parties to the relationship), or the context changes, so too should the relationship.

Table 8.7. Discussion questions when comparing relationship expectations and experience

► Are people's expectations similar? If not, why? Is differing importance attached to this aspect of the relationship? Is the context more difficult for some people? Or do they have previous negative experience?
► Are there issues where most people's expectations are notably high or low? What are the reasons for this? What are the likely consequences?
► Are people's experience similar? Again, if not, why not?
► Are there issues where most people's experience is notably high or low? What are the reasons for this? What are the likely consequences?
► Where are the biggest differences between expectations and experience? Why have expectations not been realized (eg it will take time to achieve, expectations are unrealistic, it is more difficult than expected, because of external shocks to the relationship, because one or more parties have failed to take the necessary actions)?
► How could expectations be realized?
► Overall, is the current experience of the relationship good enough to sustain health strategy and delivery?
► Do the expectations look like a reasonable target to aim for in the relationship? Do they need to be raised or lowered?

Table 8.8. Sample checklist of factors influencing relationships

Culture and value factors e.g.	Working practice factors e.g.
► Openness and honesty regarding information	► Time management
► Courtesy and respect	► Communications processes
► Basis of recognition and reward	► Consultation processes
Structural and infrastructural factors e.g.	Skills e.g.
► IT systems	► People management
► Organizational structure	► Communication skills
► Resources	► Technical knowledge/skills

Both change in the relationship and its effective operation require commitment – review without commitment may identify problems but is unlikely to lead to effective responses. Public services such as the NHS face the problem that some of their relationships are statutory or operational requirements, whether or not other parties are committed to those relationships. In such cases reviews may still be worthwhile as part of the process of identifying ways of encouraging greater commitment. Relationships are, or should be, a two-way lateral process. An important part of review should be understanding other parties' perspectives – reviews which do not address all stakeholders' expectations will be limited in their effectiveness. Finally, comes the belief that relationships can be improved and that any improvement will result in beneficial outcomes. This is perhaps of particular importance where difficult relationships are being reviewed.

Another approach designed to provide assurance of management focus rather than development support is social audit. This is based on a 'cycle of inclusion' (Fig. 8.1) which provides a regular and public assessment that key stakeholder relationships are being addressed. The cycle for any individual stakeholder may be slightly different but a number of general components are described by Wheeler and Sillanpää (1997, pp169–79). Leadership and commitment are seen as an essential precondition for an effective process which 'starts with a thorough examination of the policies, guidelines and procedures which affect the stakeholder relationships'. Determination of the scope of the audit concerns which stakeholder relationships are to be reviewed (it may not be feasible to review all initially). For larger organizations it will also include deciding which parts of the organization will initially be involved in the process.

Table 8.9. Key principles for making relationships work

1. *Accepting change.* Relationships are dynamic and therefore change is inevitable. We should accept the need to change and respond accordingly.
2. *Commitment.* The relationship between us requires time and commitment to realize its full benefits and potential.
3. *Meeting expectations.* It is important that our relationship meets my counterpart's(ies') expectations as much as my own.
4. *Relationships can be improved.* I believe that we can work together to improve this relationship.
5. *Good relationships bring benefits.* Good effective relationships are key to successful business (work) performance.

[principles 1–4 are based on the ideas of Wilmot (1987)]

Indicators are agreed with stakeholders to ensure they capture (as far as possible) their various expectations and concerns. These indicators are quantifiable outcomes or benchmarks. Determining appropriate indicators for relationships is not always easy and they can be refined as the cycle is repeated. Wheeler and Sillanpää advice, because of the importance of the process, is to at least start with something. Consultation captures the complementary soft data of satisfaction with the relationship and allows participative discussion with stakeholders. Surveys (ideally conducted by independent third parties) can complement and confirm the outcomes by enabling more people's views to be captured.

The internal audit part of the cycle consists of structured private interviews with key staff 'to explore how well individual parts of the organization are equipped to handle their stakeholder relationships'. The combination of internal and external views allows an 'account' of the relationships to be prepared. This enables managers to set objectives in response to the findings and publish these alongside the account as part of the continuing stakeholder dialogue, which continues with a repeat of the audit cycle. Where this is part of a process for building accountability in stakeholder relationships, verification is important throughout the process to ensure that the report is based on adequate participation and unbiased accurate reporting.

Relational review: sample process

A social audit (Fig. 8.1) is an extensive process which recognizes that good health is itself a process, not just a set of outcomes or measurable inputs and outputs. Reviews in the NHS will at times be large-scale organization-wide initiatives. Relational reviews should form a part of this wider process. Review, particularly when closely linked to

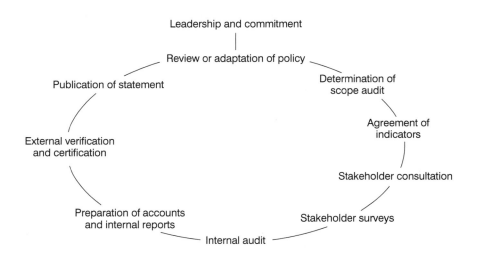

Figure 8.1. Cycle of inclusion for stakeholder relationships [Wheeler and Sillanpää (1997) p169]

development, can also be local and, in terms of resources, a much more limited process. To give an indication of how the various tools could form part of a review process a sample outline programme for the review of a 1997 NHS (Primary Care) Act pilot is set out below, based on the work of the RHC project in South Essex.

The pilot is subject to a national review of pilot sites. The local review and development support is therefore designed to focus on three key relationships or groups of relationships. These would be reviewed with particular reference to the pilot's objectives.

▶ *Practice team relationships*:
 – development of an innovative approach to teamworking
 – ensuring that teamwork and decision making within the pilot are nurse-led
 – ensuring that practice team relationships are able to support improvements in the quality of appropriate and necessary care provided to the patient population

▶ *External relationships:*
 – integration of service provision with local healthcare providers, social services, other local authority departments and voluntary groups
 – improved integration of primary and secondary care with closer working with neighbouring acute unit

▶ *Relationships with client groups*:
 – improved access to appropriate and necessary healthcare
 – improved quality of information for client groups on local services.

In each case the evaluation would look at the prioritization of relationships (in terms of operational and strategic importance, and development needs), provide initial stocktakes of specific relationships, identify priorities for relationship development and specific actions to achieve this, and review progress in the development and operation of the relationships. The latter includes reviewing whether these relationships are supporting delivery on the pilot's objectives and other relevant performance indicators.

The review process is designed to enable the development of local healthcare relationships to be evaluated against the demands of local or national initiatives (such as HImPs) as well as the pilot's specified objectives. Given the extensive range of relationships that could be included in the review process, and the possibility of changing local and national priorities during the course of the evaluation period, objectives and priorities for each stage of the review process should be confirmed before they commence.

The review follows an action research model and is based around a series of workshops held every six months. These workshops allow a cycle of planning (prioritizing relationships to be reviewed and identifying participants), action (based on the issues and actions identified in the workshops) and review (of progress made in developing relationships and the extent to which they are supporting desired outcomes). Initial participants are the practice team but can include representatives of other agencies, organizations or patient groups which were recognized as important in the review process. The timing and focus of each workshop is confirmed at each previous workshop to ensure that they focus on relevant issues and meet current development needs. A possible programme is outlined in Table 8.10.

Relational review: sample outcome

Reviewing relationships provides different outcomes from other forms of review. This is illustrated by one of the first NHS reviews we undertook: between a London health authority and a NHS community trust. The two chief executives recognized the importance of the relationship between their two organizations. Both felt that this relationship was one of their better relationships, but had only a limited picture of what the relationship was like. The review was based on a postal questionnaire sent to all individuals identified as party to the relationship – 17 at the health authority and 40 at the trust. (Incidentally, the number of people involved in the relationship proved to be greater than the participants initially expected.) This was followed up with interviews with a sample of respondents, seminars at each organization to discuss initial findings and then a joint seminar to develop an action plan.

The relationship was initially reviewed with respect to the framework of the preconditions (Table 8.5). The results of this, and subsequent initial seminars, pointed to four key issues: monitoring for value, managing change together, sharing responsibility and building reciprocal understanding (Table 8.11).

Reviewing the new NHS

The conclusions of our work on RHC in the period surrounding the launch of the new NHS can be summarized as ambiguous and ambivalent. In Chapter 10 we suggest

---

Table 8.10. Programme of workshops for relational review

Workshop 1
- ► Compare initial expectations and experience of team relationships
- ► Map external relationships

Workshop 2
- ► Include full practice team
- ► Review progress on team relationships
- ► Profile key external relationships, eg one current service delivery and one new strategic relationship
- ► Identify priorities and actions for relationship development/improvement

Workshop 3
- ► Include representatives of selected external agencies
- ► Assess extent to which relationships are enabling integrated service provision
- ► Initial stock-take of relationship with patients/user groups

Workshop 4
- ► Include representatives of user groups
- ► Review progress on service integration (including patient's perspective)
- ► Review progress on accessibility, information and quality

Workshop 5
- ► Overall review of progress against pilot objectives
- ► Review strategy for continuing service provision after pilot period and outstanding relationship development priorities

some next steps for the NHS as it continues through this transition process. In the final part of this chapter we draw together some of the conclusions from our own reviews of many parts of the NHS.

There is growing recognition of the importance of relationships for health and healthcare. They are on the agenda, both politically and in terms of health strategy, delivery and organizational development, in a way that would have been hard to

Table 8.11. Outcome of relational review between a health authority and community trust – key issues and summary of suggested actions

Key issues	To keep	To change
Monitoring for value		
Seeking robust relationship to accommodate inevitable tensions	Strong formal and informal links	Ensure both see value in providing information
Need better understanding of each other's plans and perspectives		Develop better understanding of what can be provided, eg in light of what is being provided to others
		Say if there is a problem rather than providing half-heartedly
		Seek to build good picture of a service (quality and quantity)
		Establish clearer accountability: clearly designated leads and someone with overview
Managing change together		
Perception or longer-term strategy weak: swamped by annual contracting	Collaboration over major changes	Better written records of agreements so new staff can pick up
Staff turnover could jeopardize good relationships	Retain meeting with clinicians	All agreements to be copied to relationship managers so unified updated record can be kept
		More work on joint ownership of strategy. Preface documents with key points from five-year strategy to set context
Sharing responsibility		
Different views of power in the relationship, eg over finance and accountability	Maintain the goodwill and sense of 'all in this together'	Joint risk analysis
		Honesty in good and bad news
Reciprocal understanding		
Half health authority respondents believed information from trust was not clear and easily accessible	Long-term relationships, with plenty of face-to-face contact and interchange of staff	Make more valuable – explore ways of disseminating information and understanding gained to others
Trust concerned about way information requested and lack of understanding about work pressures and infrastructural capacity		Use these meetings more efficiently: timetable and set targets
		Establish local joint early commissioning preparations
		Share organizational structures and perhaps also business plans
		More shadowing of staff

imagine four years ago. The response to this agenda has been mixed: it can be exciting, daunting and sometimes threatening. There appears to be growing impatience to move beyond rhetoric to see the substance and reality of the agenda – lasting change bringing real health improvements. It is here that ambivalence and ambiguity begin to creep in: about what kind of changes the move from rhetoric to reality will mean and whether they will on balance be an opportunity, an unsustainable burden or ineffective window dressing.

Relationships need to be actively managed: they do not just happen. If they are neglected, taken for granted or left to evolve in response to changes driven principally by other concerns, there is the considerable risk of suboptimal relationships developing. There are few short cuts to developing the relational basis for health strategy and delivery. The organizations we have worked with that are best placed to take forward the new agenda have invested considerable time and effort in building up relationships through previous organizational developments such as total purchasing pilots or consortia. Even where the basic commitment to relationships is in place, a specific focus on the relationship has revealed much that could be done further to develop and strengthen it.

The starting points are varied. Across the NHS there is a spectrum of relationships from the extremely strained and dysfunctional to the robust and highly effective. There are many factors behind this variation:

▶ the individuals involved

▶ the local history of an organization's development and the ways in which previous policies have been implemented

▶ differences in organizational cultures and leadership

▶ different local geographies

▶ different pressures on the local health system.

There would appear to be a significant danger that policy will push structures and strategies which cannot be sustained by the relationships in place and that relationship development will lag behind development in other areas.

Many healthcare relationships are changing significantly (those that have come to the fore in our work are summarized in Table 8.12) and this is creating considerable uncertainty. There is, for example, the striking four-fold increase in the number of relationships to be considered by general practice. This looks set to prompt more rigorous prioritization of relationships and consolidation to reduce the field, which will need to be complemented by better division of labour and supporting systems to aid relationships management. Maintaining all the relationships will be hard for any organization, but nigh on impossible for any individual. The characteristics of individual relationships are also changing.

These relationship changes, the transition process and the uncertainty about the real agenda combine to create a pervasive sense of ambiguity and ambivalence. One aspect of this has been role uncertainty. This applies both to professions and organizations. For GPs this may take the form of uncertainty about the future of their role as patient's advocates, in the management of primary care and in respect to other professions. For health authorities it has principally been associated with their role following the devolution of power to PCGs (and in the future Trusts). For regional offices it appears to be the squeeze between a strong centre, new regulatory mechanisms (such as NICE and the Commission for Health Improvement, or the emerging regulatory role for health authorities) and uncertainty about the prospects for regional assemblies in England. There is a competitive element to this uncertainty over, for example, professional influence or advocacy roles, which may hinder its resolution.

One consequence has been uncertain leadership. The primary care-led NHS of 1994/95 has become the NHS Executive guidance-led NHS of 1999/2000. In places we have witnessed temporary leadership vacuums surrounding the establishment of PCGs: sometimes because of a reluctance to assume leadership for fear of alienating others – there was no consensus as to where leadership properly lay; sometimes as a result of disempowerment – fearful for personal futures, forced to abandon previous organizational initiatives and reverting to dependency on the centre. The appropriate style of leadership has also changed. There has been a premium on inclusive leadership to manage the transition, as opposed to the entrepreneurial leadership which has championed new initiatives in the past.

An important task of leadership will be to generate trust and confidence, to articulate

---

Table 8.12. Changing characteristics of healthcare relationships

NHS to population/community/individual patient
► Attempt to balance rights and responsibilities
► Primary care role in public health increasingly focused at community level
► Greater accountability of NHS to local communities
► Modernized relationship emphasizing inclusiveness, openness and accessibility
► Individual patient-professional relationship remains at the heart of system, but tension with community focus and new non-relationship based services (eg walk in centres)

NHS to government
► Politicized service may create uneasy three-way relationship between government, NHS and public
► NHS and government competing as advocates of quality and patients' interests
► Need to build relationships of trust and confidence

Primary care organizations to health authorities
► Health authority becoming custodian/guarantor/regulator of relationships in local health economy
► Initial tensions between development and emerging regulatory role
► Relinquishing control to emerging primary care trusts will not always be easy

NHS and local government
► For many a new relationship
► Limited mutual understanding, with significant cultural and organizational differences
► NHS uncertain how to resource this relationship
► Organizational basis for local integration not yet clear – few models in practice

Interprofessional relationships
► New breed of 'primary healthcare workers' may develop
► Continuing conflict over professional interests

Inter-practice relationships
► Financial implications uncertain
► Clinical governance and shared accountability

and sell the benefits and opportunities of the new NHS, and to model and promote the behaviours that it requires. Trust and confidence are the antidote to uncertainty about roles; personal, professional and organizational prospects and the policy agenda. They are also necessary in integrating the innovation and the monitoring of the quality agenda. They are an essential prerequisite for securing the engagement and commitment that 'modernizing' the NHS requires. In the absence of such trust and confidence the currency of change must be tangible benefits and improvements, not just a vision of the future. Effective leaders of PCGs, for example, have identified specific benefits such as improved back pain services (and ensured that they are realized), which have enabled the better integration of reluctant fringe practices.

Leadership in the new NHS will also need to model appropriate behaviours. This is important because some of the cultural changes required are significant. Parts of this may include rekindling the spirit of public service as a unifying theme for the NHS and its partners in public health. A lack of commonality has been one of the major obstacles to relationships that we have encountered. Tactically this can be countered by finding common enemies, through city-wide initiatives or identifying shared benefits. But something deeper than this is needed. The meaning of the stated unifying themes of equity or quality has corroded: it can perhaps be recaptured but the concept of public service may prove to be a richer seam of shared values and objectives.

The NHS is in transition. There is no way back – indeed there is no golden age to which to go back. If the modernization of the NHS does not mean creating the right relationships between the NHS and the nation, between public services and government, and between health care organizations and professions, then it will have failed to establish a key part of the new NHS foundations. Experience is currently mixed: the agenda, ambiguous; the commitment, ambivalent. We have seen exciting indications of what the new NHS could become. We have also seen much that indicates that there are many birth pains ahead. In Chapters 9 and 10 we specifically address the future quality and prospects of the health system in the UK and suggest some next steps to aid this transition.

Summary

Review should be both forward and backward looking, supporting each of the previous functions and linking them together. Relationships should not be neglected. Appropriate tools, tailored to the wide range of questions that can be asked about healthcare relationships, are now being developed. In reviewing the developing relationships of the new NHS we have found considerable diversity, ambiguity and ambivalence. The changing relational map has created uncertainty about roles, the real agenda and leadership. Trust and confidence need to be built and real unifying themes identified if modernization is to create the right relationships between the NHS and the nation, between public services and government and between healthcare organizations and professions; these will be a key part of the new NHS foundations.

References

Berne E (1968). *Games People Play: The Psychology of Human Relationships*. Harmondsworth: Penguin.

Bion W (1961). *Experience in Groups*. London: Tavistock.

Devlin M (1998). *Primary Health Care and the Public Sector*. Oxford: Radcliffe Medical Press.

Hinde R (1997). *Relationships: A Dialectical Perspective*. Hove: Psychology Press.

Hudson R (1998). *Primary Care and Social Care*. Leeds: Nuffield Institute.

Iles V (1997). *Really Managing Health Care.* Buckingham: Open University Press.

Meads G (1997). *Power and Influence in the NHS*. Radcliffe Medical Press, Oxford: 29.

Meads G (1998). Integrated primary care: the relational challenge. *Journal of Integrated Care* **2**: 51–4.

NHS Executive (1997). *PMS Pilots under the NHS (Primary Care) Act 1997. A Guide to Local Evaluation,* 97PP0130. Leeds: Primary Care Division.

NHS Executive (1998) Consultation document of Performance Framework.

Peckham S, Taylor P, Macdonald J *et al* (1986). *Towards a Public Health Model of Primary Care*. Birmingham: The Public Health Trust.

West M and Pillinger T (1996). *An Evaluation of Teambuilding in Primary Care*. London: Health Education Authority.

Wheeler D and Sillanpää M (1997). *The Stakeholder Corporation*. London: Pitman Publishing: 169–79.

Wilmot W (1987). *Dyadic Communication*. London: Random House.

9
Quality

'As a dream comes when there are many cares,
so the speech of a fool when there are many words.'
(Ecclesiastes 5: 3)

A flexible friend

For those engaged in defining policy over the past 10 years, no term has been more convenient or malleable than that of 'quality'. While it would not quite be fair to say that it can mean all things to all people in the NHS, it certainly has been the case during the past decade that different interest groups in the UK health system have found it in their interest to use 'quality' as the banner under which their range of sometimes very different causes can be best promoted. The pursuit of quality, accordingly, was used to help justify the arrival of successful private sector entrepreneurs and advocates on NHS boards in the early 1990s, when the NHS internal market was introduced. Quality (and 'choice') for a while then became virtually synonymous with the 'consumerist' tendency in the official NHS glossary of terms; many a senior nurse survived in an executive role by being reinvented as a 'Director of Quality'. Quality as a concept in practice has in effect been up for grabs. To define it effectively is to exert a significant degree of control in and over contemporary health and healthcare developments.

This has become crystal clear over the past two years as the leading politicians of the new NHS have taken control of the concept. It is now the turn of New Labour to define what quality means. As a result, during the four-year period of the Relational Health Care (RHC) project, we have witnessed a faster growth in government-derived communications on this subject than any other. Over the same period, however, this is also the subject on which we have observed and felt the widest gulf between the central enthusiasm and local response. The latter, in our experience, often remains flat and sometimes suspicious, particularly amongst the traditional health providers and authorities of the mainstream NHS. Even those whose remits include the stated aim of uniting the 'New NHS' are regarded as not yet quite trustworthy, especially when they have such infinitely flexible friends as 'quality' and seem likely in their pronounce-ments to preface yet another significant shift in the balance of power within the health system.

Table 9.1 illustrates the pivotal role and political significance of the new approach to quality. It was the first slide used by senior civil servants in the 1997/98 period in public presentations on the 'key messages' of the new NHS. Quality was described as one of the new 'unifying concepts' along with 'integration' and 'efficiency', and each was applied at individual, service and organizational levels. The stated strategy of the

Table 9.1. The new NHS: key messages (Source: Capita and KPMG National Conferences on the New NHS, Spring 1997)

▶ Themes:
  addressing inequity,
  improving quality,
  increasing efficiency
▶ Underpinned by:
  making the NHS a better place to work
▶ And so:
  restoring public confidence in the NHS

---

government was to 'ensure that quality of care becomes the driving force for the development of health services in England', through clear and consistent national standards backed up by effective monitoring systems and local delivery mechanisms (NHS Executive 1998, pp2–3). Clinical governance is the new flagship cresting the waves of this new quality movement. Teamwork, lifelong learning, evidence-based medicine, and user and carer involvement are just some of the crew members.

In the central guidance on clinical governance, no fewer than 34 separate roles and responsibilities are set out for every level in the NHS, with 14 of these to be delivered by the new primary care organizations (Table 9.2). The captain of the ship is the National Institute for Clinical Excellence (NICE). It is here that the responsibility for detecting and dealing with poor performance and adverse events ultimately comes to rest. It is this role, aligned with the new powers attributed to primary care groups (PCGs) and primary care trusts (PCTs), which is causing much of the unease. The original consultation documents of The New NHS spoke of generating a completely 'new culture' organization-wide within restored NHS structures over a 10-year period of 'modernization' (NHS Executive 1997). The aim was a 'first class service' (Department of Health 1998). Much of the experience of the first two years has been the other way around: an 'old' culture of central political control and GP hegemony is being restored, while further organization-wide structural experiments are tried of which PCGs and NICE are simply the most manifest illustrations.

Where has this left quality? The impression of an ambiguous concept once more provoking ambivalent reactions arises because the relationships are not (yet anyway) there to sustain genuine quality as a thematic of the whole healthcare system – which, of course, in relational terms is what quality needs to be. The theory is now in place. The studies of accreditation, in particular, have meant that quality can be applied to the process of converting inputs to outputs, and sometimes even outcomes, through meas-

---

Table 9.2. Clinical governance: primary care responsibilities [based on NHS Executive (1998), pp12–13]

▶ Rules of new primary care organisation: Management accountability for practice of constituent parts within PCG/PCT
  →
▶ Joint management accountability with relevant others for externally provided services
  →
▶ Inclusion within all commissioning arrangements/agreements
▶ Priority application for internal and external development programmes

---

ures for a wide range of linked components in this process (eg Scrivens 1995). There are protocols and guidelines for clinical practice, standards for health and safety, a range of audit mechanisms for organizational procedures; surveys to test public satisfaction and charters to establish public expectations, etc. Quality now has a fully usable toolkit and as a result the NHS has an unprecedented range of both external inspectors and internal 'quality' programmes with continuous improvement as their theme. Quality is no longer systematic and separate, but potentially at least systemic and comprehensive; and as such it is a corporate issue. Chief executives and NHS boards can now be expected to assume organizational accountabilities for quality. The theory is ready; it has been translated into policy and pilots. The practice now awaits.

The professional paradox

The policy is unequivocal that the NHS professionals will have the 'lead' role in this practice: doctors and nurses. This is framed as a declaration of confidence. Local professionals will deserve the support and sanction of national quality frameworks. The New NHS white paper sets the tone:

> 'Local doctors and nurses, who best understand patients' needs will shape services. Patients will be guaranteed national standards of excellence so that they can have confidence in the quality of the services they receive. There will be new incentives and new sanctions to improve quality and efficiency.'
>
> (Secretary of State for Health 1997, p5)

It could hardly be clearer or more assertive:

> 'The new NHS will have quality at its heart.'
>
> (Secretary of State for Health 1997, p17)

So why have we found so much ambivalence? Why are NHS staff still suspicious of the intent? Why indeed do some of the medical professionals we have encountered see in 'quality' the seeds of their own self-destruction? Why is this true even in the new primary care organizations where we could expect to see clinical governance embraced as a vital part of their new commissioning armour: essential for getting to grips with both recalcitrant practices and traditionally separatist secondary care providers? The answer appears to lie in the translation from 'profession' to 'professionalism' and the tensions between 'generalist' and 'expert' that are occurring as a result of how the 'quality' concept is being applied in practice (Fisher 1999). The effect of these changes is further to disturb the basic relationships of the healthcare system. Whether by design or default, individual and collective identities are less secure and the future direction seems uncertain. It is not a 'quality' environment.

Professions in the UK, and especially the medical profession, have enjoyed connotations of elevated social and financial status often not experienced in other countries. As Europe extends to include several former 'Eastern bloc' countries, for example, we realize that it was quite possible for a viable national healthcare system to operate with 'lead' professionals whose salaries would not even come halfway up UK pay ladders. For general practice, as for medical consultants in the

UK, this has been inconceivable in the past. Social and financial status has been part of the package of being in a profession; along with clinical autonomy, self-regulatory rights and a certain knowledge base. No wonder the ultimate sense of loyalty has been to the profession itself.

But in the new NHS the principal allegiance is now expected to be somewhere else. Here again a 179 majority in parliament makes a massive difference. The political imperative is for the organization itself (as a proxy for the public and patient) to be where fundamental loyalties lie. We must all own and own up to the 'New NHS'. Clinical and corporate governance are required accountabilities at the level of NHS boards, into which the professions are now incorporated. Six or seven of the 11 or 12 members of PCG boards are, after all, usually GPs, with two from the nursing profession also at the table. As a result it is representatives of the professions themselves – elected by their peers – who are set up to be responsible for challenging clinical autonomy, putting a cap on financial aspirations, adjusting employment status and above all restricting and augmenting rights of self-regulation; all in the name of 'quality'. It is like dismantling a long-held, much-cherished persona.

In its place goes 'professionalism'. This has rather different connotations from that of the 'profession'. Professionalism is essentially about the way the task is undertaken. Accordingly, into this 'process' definition goes interprofessional collaboration, new skills mixes, externally verifiable standards, a wider range of qualifications and the demonstrable use of standards. Quality through 'professionalism', unlike the 'professions', can be applied to all. It encourages a wider sense of vocation and includes within its scope both technical and non-medical skills. It is a much more flexible concept and one which offers the prospect of being much more affordable in practice.

The new tensions between 'generalist' and 'expert' are travelling along the same path. Having been marginal for so long, the expert is now moving into the mainstream of decision-making responsibilities within the new NHS. The inspectors of the Commission for Health Improvement (CHI) and NICE are the most visible illustrations; their power and influence growing as that of NHS general management diminishes. To a significant extent the roles and responsibilities of the latter are transferring to other generalists: the GPs at the head of the new primary care organizations. But this is no simple swap. The conversion process sees PCGs required to take on decisions about priorities for services and expenditure not simply from within their traditional context of holistic personal care, but rather with the requirements to:

- ▶ comply with clinical indicators derived from medical researchers
- ▶ meet the disease management targets set by specialists and public health consultants
- ▶ conform to the performance indices drawn up by financial and organizational auditors
- ▶ use the communications networks devised by the gurus of IM&T.

Quality lies in expertise and quality is now at the head of the table.

In an increasingly intricate, complex and sophisticated healthcare system, the 'generalist' and his or her philosophy can easily seem vulnerable and under attack. We have found that this sense of threat pervades many of those in PCGs, particularly in areas such as Wolverhampton, Enfield and Camden where there has been very little experience of general management in primary care. Where such experience has been developed, for example through the total purchasing pilots in Wakefield, Runcorn and Woking, we have witnessed a stronger capacity to develop quality from within, embracing both new expertise and the new 'professionalism'. As we enter the year 2000, however, these examples remain the exceptions not the rule.

Primary care perspectives

For most GPs it still feels as though quality has slipped in through the back door. Even their leading 'quality' advocate, Sir Donald Irvine, has been unswerving in his support for exclusive self-regulation. In defining the 'practice of quality' the term is only deployed explicitly to what Irvine identifies as the new core general practice function of secondary care commissioning; only covertly to the cycle of audit, research, education and development (Irvine and Irvine 1996); and not directly to the provision of General Medical Practice itself.

It has been particularly important to tread warily in introducing the idea to primary care in the UK itself. Figure 9.1 illustrates the reasons for this caution. It is hardly any time at all since simply being a GP was seen as a secure quality safeguard. The qualification was enough. Experience added to this automatically and was recognized contractually and financially in the seniority payments system of the 1966–89 period. The introduction of medical audit in the early 1990s, under Sir Donald Irvine's tutelage, made scarcely a dent in this image. The audit was a private, GP-to-GP affair, as were the new associated arrangements for their postgraduate education. The power was still with the profession and the rights of the Family Health Services Authorities, right up until their demise in 1995, were restricted simply to registering that the audits and the training programmes had taken place.

Suddenly, in the space of little more than four years, there is clinical governance: quality requirements at corporate and individual levels for GPs and legally incorporated, via PCGs' formal accountabilities, into their terms of service. Hardly had clinical audits tentatively got under way with other professionals, on such 'safe' topics as asthma management and protocols for diabetic care, than the potential sledgehammer of quality as (political) scrutiny came into force. For a sector whose frontline is so richly varied that the 'multiple, overlapping and at times, mutually exclusive perspectives which do not lend themselves to any unifying paradigm (for) the concept of quality' (Greenhalgh and Eversley 1999, p3) are more evident than anywhere else in the health care environment, the speed and abruptness of the developments has been disarming. Greenhalgh and Eversley's (1999, p58) guiding principles for the development of quality indicators – local definition by those who will be assessed through to 'deep learning' processes that fundamentally reframe behaviour – are at least being placed at risk if not to one side.

As a result current primary care perspectives are not positive. The meaning of quality has changed within a decade from a check on the size of a consulting room to

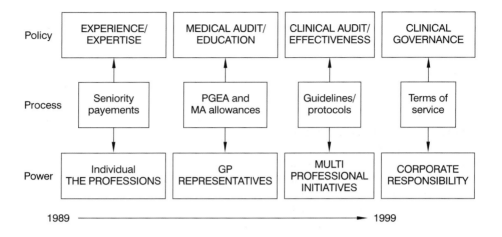

Fig. 9.1. (Service) Quality in primary care

the efficiency and effectiveness of the consultation itself. GPs who are now expected to question the clinical and organizational quality of others have yet to answer the new questions about their own services' quality. Such is the speed of the change that it is a schizophrenic relationship. Accordingly and not surprisingly, we have attended a number of early PCG meetings (eg West Haringey and West Surrey) where GP members have appeared only too willing to pass on the 'lead' clinical governance role to one of the other professional representatives, or even the lay member. To many it has tasted like the poisoned chalice, putting at risk the preservation and future prospects of primary care.

Temporal theologies

The modern 'quality' movement in the NHS has often reminded us of a religious movement. Those who developed the original tenets of modern 'quality' [eg Berwick (1993), Donabedian (1966)] are often referred to as 'spiritual gurus' from 'across the water', ie the US. We have sometimes heard those who support their ideas described as 'followers' or 'disciples', and more broadly, the NHS itself over the past 10 years has not infrequently adopted and adapted quasi-Biblical language to express its reforming zeal. Hence 'mission' has become a management term, 'trust' turned into the name of an organization and 'sharing' used as a euphemism for either surrendering resources or revealing a weakness. What was precious has been turned into the common place. Profoundly fundamental values have been devalued. That 'quality' has become some-thing of a modern god in the NHS, and of course in other public service and private enterprise systems, says something about the power of the traditional healthcare professions which quality is now being used to circumvent and constrain. It also highlights the resourcefulness of political leaderships in terms of exerting power when continuous structural change limits their options for control. More important, however, is what it signifies for behaviour and relationships. The family of 'quality' value concepts can be seen to constitute a temporal theology designed to influence attitudes and control conduct to politically determined organizational ends in ways that religions have historically used to shape personal ethics and their expression. To some extent this juxtaposition seems only possible because of the demise of those religions and, in particular, the increasingly minority popular status of Christianity. No wonder that the sense of ambivalence is profound.

These feelings are often the toughest to come to terms with for those who are the busiest. In the NHS this certainly applies to practice managers, community nurses and those working in the big hospitals of central London. They hardly have time to identify let alone articulate and resolve the ambiguities in the policies, such as those emanating from 'quality', that impinge upon their congested routines. Over the past two years in such overloaded parts of the NHS as these, Iles has taught to great effect her creed of generosity and discipline as the way for individual healthcare professionals to manage qualitatively in their hard-pressed local circumstances and roles (Table 9.3). The list begins and ends with the right sort of relationships, first for internal and finally for external quality results. Her approach has clearly helped those in, for example, the new primary care organizations of Ealing, Lambeth and East London, because the qualities she lists are in touch both with where her audiences are personally and with the essentially personal nature of the healthcare they deliver every day.

Ultimately quality is a political and organizational value. Fundamentally it has personal, social and spiritual values that apply to health and healthcare. These have always been, and will always be, the permanent sources of the relationships with patients and the public, and it is those at the point-of-contact with the latter, especially we have found in primary care, who recognize this best. Sometimes this recognition understandably is unconscious. Nevertheless it is still powerful and as such it is an effective antidote to the otherwise all embracing reaches of the quality movement and its disciples.

Accordingly, the lesson is that quality is an expedient value. It is vital to understand who controls its definition, how this is decided, where this definition is applied and whether or not this is appropriate. Its natural habitat is the alternative society of websites and commodities, of fax modems and the Internet, where the key relation-

Table 9.3. Features of a culture of generosity and discipline: the lubricant in healthcare organizations [based on Iles (1997), pp105–6]

- ▶ High quality, robust relationships throughout the organization
- ▶ Systems which work with rather than against human nature
- ▶ Everyone receiving all the information they need (but not more)
- ▶ Modelling of behaviour (organizational leaders) want to see in others, including 'rising above' quarrels
- ▶ The selling not solving of problems by management
- ▶ Abandoning practices which inhibit the development of confidence in junior staff
- ▶ Enhancing self respect
- ▶ Developing healthy collaborative relationships with all other stakeholders in quality outcomes

ships are those of information technology. As a value quality cannot enduringly shape healthcare because it fundamentally is a myriad of personal, not clinical or organizational, contacts and relationships. For these personal contacts relational values are required. Secular sources cannot supply them effectively and certainly not on a lasting basis. Quality, therefore, produces mixed reactions from the zeal of converts to the alienation of cynics. For relationships it is a minefield and certainly not a panacea for reconciling long-term different and divergent interests. For the NHS, as for other public services, the way forward lies not attempting to create its own new 'absolutes', but in ensuring that its new professionals, local resource managers, partnerships and primary care organizations are those which best allow individuals and communities to express their personal connections and their relationship needs through the vehicles of delivering effective healthcare and promoting better health.

In the contemporary NHS and contemporary society such a scenario can seem both elusive and fragile. It is to these future prospects that we finally turn our attention. If the prospects for a genuinely relationship-based health system are to become stronger, then it is essential that the values which do support it are much stronger than that of quality and their products much less transient. Above all, it is essential for the NHS in transition that these values have the real means of turning policy into practice. Otherwise we will be left with a policy seen as too good for the NHS to deliver and future prospects too dismal to countenance.

Summary

The politics of the contemporary NHS have often been played out through the different meanings afforded the concept of quality. This has led to a lack of both clarity and certainty in reactions to its latest incarnation in respect of clinical care and its organization. There are risks to relationships in healthcare arising from the use of quality principles to justify stronger central scrutiny. Suspicion will not be allayed if quality is credited with a false moral value, when it is the ethics of personal and social relationships which are, and should remain, fundamental to healthcare.

References

Berwick D (1991). Curing Health Care: New Strategies for Quality Improvement, Josey Bass, San Francisco.

Department of Health (1998). A First Class Service, HSC 1998/113. London: Department of Health.

Donabedian A (1966). Evaluating the quality of medical care. Millbank Memorial Fund Quarterly 44: 166–203.

Fisher E (1999). Professionalism and Expertise in the Public Services: a Historical and Conceptual Overview. Southampton: University of Southampton.

Greenhalgh T and Eversley J (1999). Quality in General Practice. London: Kings Fund Publishing.

Iles V (1997). Really Managing Health Care. Buckingham: Open University Press.

Irvine D and Irvine S (1996). The Practice of Quality. Oxford: Radcliffe Medical Press: 25.

NHS Executive (1998). Quality in the new NHS, 15355. Wetherby: Department of Health Wetherby: 2–3.

NHS Executive (1997). Education and Training Planning Guidance, EL (97) 58. Leeds: NHS Executive.

Scrivens E (1995). Accreditation, Protecting the Professional or the Consumer? Buckingham: Open University Press.

Secretary of State for Health (1997). The New NHS: Modern, Dependable, Cm 3807. London: HMSO.

10
Prospects

*'All share a common destiny – the righteous and the wicked,
the good and the bad, the clean and the unclean, those who
offer sacrifices and those who do not.'*
(Ecclesiastes 9: 2)

The multiplier

The pages that have paved the way for this final chapter have described changing relationships in contemporary healthcare which amount to both fundamental opportunities for growth and profound risks of implosion, especially for the institution of the NHS – at one and the same time. It is tempting, in our concluding comments to say simply that explaining and understanding the source of the themes of ambivalence and ambiguity, to which we have repeatedly returned in our account, is enough. Awareness and recognition of the real issues are usually regarded, in therapeutic terms, as a large part of the solution to the problem. For some of the components of the health system we have addressed – quality, for example – this may be true; but for most of the others (eg policy, development, review), to assert that the answers simply lie in intellectual comprehension or even empathic understanding would be to 'bottle out'. For readers and writers alike it would be a frustrating way to finish.

It would also be to miss the point. For the NHS in transition, if we are to know how to bridge the gap between policy intention and practice implementation, tangible responses are required. The NHS is experiencing a massive multiplication in its relationships requirements as a result of the New NHS policy developments. On paper this is no bad thing. In practice what so severely jeopardizes the prospects of it becoming a good thing is that NHS personnel, by dint of recent conditioning in their jobs, and owing to the diminution of their relational skills and experience outside of work in today's technological society (see Baker 1996), may simply be unable to cope with the scale and complexities of contemporary healthcare relationships. They are often, as we have witnessed, hopelessly ill equipped to do so. In this respect, of course, they are no different from those working to 'new' policies in many other parts of the politically-driven public services sector.

The tangibles

This analysis represents a pessimistically negative prospect. What could be the practical vision to turn this around, based on some of the lessons of our analysis? How has our period of participant observation affected the agenda set out at the start of the action research cycle in Chapter 1? What, in short, now represent the genuinely positive prospects (Table 10.1)?

First, there is the prospect of the NHS moving from a centralized, national public institution based on such political values as quality and equity to a nationwide service of (say 500) community organizations bound together by such relational values as parity, acceptance and proximity. It seems vital that this is the vision for the next 'Level 5' stage of NHS organizational development; not just for primary care trusts (PCTs), but for other major healthcare providers and commissioners as well.

Secondly, as the above suggests, the main providers in the health system must be rehabilitated and regenerated as rich sources of relational healthcare. To write them off as either stigmatizing or depersonalizing institutions run by clinical hierarchies is both intellectually lazy and morally unfair. It is also, in terms of establishing the new NHS, deeply destructive. The district general, university and local community hospitals of this country remain very capable of mounting fiercely effective resistance movements. The perception of secondary care providers of the NHS, and many of those outside the NHS, needs to be reframed so that they are seen not as at best separate communities, but as *of* the local communities with much more robust representational and resourcing arrangements to demonstrate their local ownership. The future model is not that of the old district health authority but one that gathers together the lessons for local ownership of successful housing associations, schools and modern charities. Perceived in this way they can cease to be regarded as the end-of-the-line for rationing decisions, from which they are now increasingly excluded; but rather one of the key starting points for setting priorities as genuine participants with a parity 'stakeholding' in the local NHS community organizations.

To convert this from perception into reality requires a third substantive shift, this time in terms of responsibilities for the public resourcing of a nationwide, universal NHS to local levels. Already for the NHS in transition it is crystal clear to experienced political commentators that the sort of relationships required to take us where we want to get to cannot be created through an escalation in operational and policy guidance from a central political administration (eg Robinson 1998, Riddell 1999). This produces too much dependency. It empowers the Civil Service but not the citizen.

> *'It is an illusion to fancy that an organisation that is internally unrelational can deliver an effective relational service.'*
>
> (Hitchings 1999)

Table 10.1. The new NHS: six tangible ways forward

- ► Locally owned NHS organizations with relational values
- ► Reframing NHS providers in and of communities
- ►   Compatible NHS local resourcing and relationship responsibil
- ►   Process-oriented performance management valuing relational differen
- ►   Relationship-based education and training cul
- ► Restored role of public institution as a source of society

The right sort of relationships in tomorrow's health system, where primary care organizations are the pivotal points of performance, requires service and financial responsibilities to go hand in hand and to reside with the same set of local decision-making relationships. This is the price of striving for equity.

Performance in this context is broadening its meaning. The fourth tangible product of a more relationally-oriented health system must recognize this in its monitoring arrangements. Partnerships can be profiled; the means are there to audit relationships within and across organizations and against specific policy objectives, and even to develop new objectives. The components of relational proximity (see Table 4.1), for example, can be scored. It is perfectly possible to quantify over time the progress or otherwise of collaboration and cooperation whether it be across health action zones or in a healthy living centre; and to incorporate the assessments in frameworks for review that include the customary financial, clinical and activity indicators. Indeed, to do so is vital for the preservation of a national health service with nationally administered safeguards and guarantees of equivalent patient access, clinical standards and service levels across the country. Without these measures 'the proper coordination of commissioning' upon which 'long term NHS Service Agreements' depend will be jeopardized (Department of Health 1998). The government needs to be able to show that it feels all right for local people to relate to different, even divergent, healthcare systems in (broadly) the same way, with (broadly) the same results. Otherwise, ironically, new primary care organizations could spell the end of the decentralized new NHS.

We have learnt that too often monitoring and development have become divorced. The fifth tangible is about their reconciliation through relationship-based education and training approaches. In particular, the need for interprofessional curricula content and interactive learning processes has been highlighted. We have learnt, however, that this will not happen simply through exhortation or even disseminating the learning from local good practice which is simply too few and far between. A national programme for 'training the trainers' is required. The Deans and Pro-Vice Chancellors (Health) need to be taken to one side; the continuation audit criteria for university postgraduate programmes need to be revised and the standard NHS contractual terms for commissioning consultancy and facilitation completely overhauled. Together this amounts to a significant strategy for cultural change.

Love

Sixthly, the new NHS can move out this sense of being in constant transition by responding to the peculiar opportunity presented by a government at least partly in sympathy with the Christian Socialist tradition of remembering what is the fundamental role of a public institution. Public bodies must clearly adjust to their contemporary circumstances through their changing policies, strategies and structures. We have argued that they can, and should, do so in ways that convert the emphasis on better relationships for health into new forms of practice which engage with many people and sectors not previously regarded as part of the NHS. This extension of influence could be seen as a serious risk – diluting and diffusing the traditional NHS through, for example, the mixed status of new primary care organizations (see Table 5.3). We would argue, rather, that the key messages from our period of participant observation in the new NHS points to influence extending in a different direction.

Overall, there is now the opportunity to restore what the NHS has to offer as one of the most significant public agencies for binding together civil society at national, regional and local levels. As such the NHS is a most precious resource for strengthening relationships within communities and across local and regional boundaries. The sixth and final tangible opportunity lies, accordingly, in recalling that the NHS is the way in which as a society we demonstrate our care for our neighbour: how, indeed, we fulfil the ancient commandment to love our neighbour as ourselves.

Summary

The shortfalls in NHS relationships serve as the major obstacle to successful implementation of ambitious policies for improving health and healthcare. Nevertheless, expectations of these relationships continue to expand. Positive action is therefore essential. Six practical ways forward are described. Together these are aimed at returning the NHS to its original role and meaning as a fundamental form of fellowship for both our local and national communities.

References

Baker N, ed (1996). *Building a Relational Society*. Aldershot: Arena.
Department of Health (1999). *Commissioning in the New NHS. Commissioning Services 1999–2000*, HSC 1998/198. Wetherby: Department of Health.
Hitchings M (1999). New managerialism or new relationships. *Relational Justice Bulletin* **3**: 6–7.
Riddell P (1999). Beyond the Tony and John show. *Public Finance* **July**: 16–18.
Robinson R (1998). The new NHS: primary care groups as managed care organisations. In: Shelton R and Williamson V, eds. *Fifty Years of the NHS: Continuities and Discontinuities in Health Policy*. Brighton: University of Brighton: 58–71.

Appendix A:
Relational Health Care Project Participants

RHC Project Advisory Board Members, 1995–99

Geoffrey Meads, Professor of Health Services Development, Health Management Group, City University, London (Chair)
Duncan Vere, Professor (Emeritus) of Therapeutics, University of London (Vice-Chair)
John Buckler, Retired Senior Lecturer/Consultant Paediatrician, Leeds General Infirmary
Mary Gobbi, Senior Lecturer, Nursing School, Southampton University
Derrick Hill, Head of Strategic Development, East Norfolk Health Authority
Jenny Griffiths, Chief Executive, West Surrey Health Authority
Jeff James, Chief Executive, Gloucestershire Health Authority
Michael Schluter, Director, Relationships Foundation
Keith Whale, Regional Manager, Merck, Sharpe and Dohme

RHC Project Staff Team, 1995–99

John Ashcroft, Research Director
Tom Robson, Project Manager
Cathy Lewis, Project Officer
Coralie Susans, Researcher
Karen Goddard, Graduate Assistant

RHC Project Sites, 1995–99

Members of over 150 primary care organizations and 30 health authorities/boards in England, Wales and Scotland have used RHC materials, including primary care groups in the following districts/localities since 1 April 1998:
Aldershot
Andover
Camden and Islington
East Wiltshire
Fife
Leeds
Lincolnshire
Newham
North Wales

Nottingham
Oldham
Somerset
South Essex
Southampton and South West Hampshire
Suffolk
Tyneside
West Surrey
Winchester
Wolverhampton

RHC Conferences, 1995–99

In addition to six national conferences/workshops hosted by the Relationships Foundation, the following organizations have included RHC contributions at their events:
Association of Managers in General Practice (1997)
Capita (1997–98)
Harrogate Public Sector Management Centre (1998)
Institute of Health Services Management (1997)
NHS Staff College, Wales (1997–98)
Health Education Authority (1998–99)
European Multi-Professional Education Network (1998).

RHC Discussion Groups (1998)

A. Caring

Dr John Buckler, Retired Senior Lecturer/Consultant Paediatrician, Leeds General Infirmary
Dr Eunice Burton, Retired Consultant Gynaecologist
Ms Janet Cox, Snr Lecturer in Nursing, University of Luton
Dr Andrew Fergusson, General Secretary, Christian Medical Fellowship
Ms Michelle Turner, Health Visitor, Riverside Community Healthcare Trust
Professor Duncan Vere, Professor (Emeritus) of Therapeutics, University of London

B. Collaboration

Mr Alan Carpenter, East Wiltshire Healthcare NHS Trust
Mr Ian Hammond, Bedfordshire and Shires Health and Care Trust
Mr Derrick Hill, East Norfolk Health Authority
Dr June Huntington, Birmingham University
Dr Michael Sheldon, Department of General Practice and Primary Care, St Bartholomew's Hospital
Ms Lynn Smith, Centre For Advancement of Inter-professional Education
Ms Jenny Stepheny, Independent Consultant
Mr Ted Unsworth, ex-Director of Social Services

C. Competition

Ms Karen Ashton, East Wiltshire Community Trust
Dr Tim Billington, Lordshill Health Centre
Mr David Coleman, Community Pharmacist, Southampton
Ms Rachel Graham, Royal London Hospital
Ms Karen Gurnhill, Lambeth, Southwark and Lewisham Health Authority
Ms Ann Jones, Trinity Care
Mr Steve Lawrence, Westminster Health Care
Mr Ian Piper, Portsmouth Healthcare NHS Trust
Mr Mervin Suffield, Trinity Care
Ms Kate Wortham, Independent Consultant

For further details on any of the above please contact John Ashcroft, Research Director, Relationships Foundation, 3 Hooper Street, Cambridge, CB1 2NZ.

Appendix B:
Relational Health Care Project Papers and Publications

The Relationships Foundation (1996). *Relational Health Care*, preliminary report for discussion purposes. Copies available from 3 Hooper Street, Cambridge, CB1 2NZ.

Robson T (1997). *NHS/Social Services Relationships*, report on feasibility project funded by King's Fund. Cambridge: Relationships Foundation.

Susans C (1997). *Stress, Disease and Social Support*. Unpublished research paper, Relationships Foundation, Cambridge.

Lewis C (1997). Enhancing collaboration in primary care. *Primary Care* **7**(10): 5–6.

Meads G (1998). Integrated primary care: the relational challenge. *Journal of Integrated Care* **2**: 51–4.

The Jubilee Centre (1998). *Biblical Perspectives on Health and Health Care Relationships*. Copies available from 3 Hooper Street, Cambridge CB1 2NZ.

Coleman D (1998). *A Relational Perspective on Medicine Taking*. Unpublished paper in support of PhD submission, Portsmouth University.

Benaim R (1999). Front line workers. *British Journal of Health Care Management* **5**(Suppl) 2–5.

Meads G (1999). Research matrix reveals typology of primary care groups. *British Journal of Health Care Management* **5**(3): 96–100.

Meads G, Killoran A, Ashcroft J, Cornish Y (1999). *Mixing Oil and Water*. London: HEA Publications.

Meads G and Ashcroft J (2000). *Relationships in the NHS*. London: RSM Publications.

Relational Health Care Project Updates (1995–2000). Relationships Foundation. Copies from 3 Hooper Street, Cambridge CB1 2NZ.

Publications arising from other Relationships Foundations programmes include:

Schluter M and Lee D(1993). *The 'R' Factor*. London: Hodder & Stoughton.

Burnside J and Baker N, eds (1994). *Relational Justice*. Winchester: Waterside Press.

Baker N, ed (1996). *Building a Relational Society*. Aldershot : Arena.

'Of making many books there is no end,
and much study wearies the body'
(Ecclesiastes 12: 12)

Index